Ageing and Health in India

Editors

C. Shanthi Johnson

S. Irudaya Rajan

RAWAT PUBLICATIONS

Jaipur • New Delhi • Bangalore • Hyderabad • Guwahati

ISBN 81-316-0281-8

Published by
Prem Rawat for **Rawat Publications**
Satyam Apts, Sector 3, Jawahar Nagar, Jaipur 302 004 (India)
Phone: 0141 265 1748 / 7006 Fax: 0141 265 1748
E-mail: info@rawatbooks.com
Website: www.rawatbooks.com

New Delhi Office
4858/24, Ansari Road, Daryaganj, New Delhi 110 002
Phone: 011 2326 3290

Also at *Bangalore, Hyderabad* and *Guwahati*

Typeset by Rawat Computers, Jaipur
Printed at Chaman Enterprises, New Delhi

Contents

Preface

"Respect your father and your mother, so that you may live a long time in the land that I am giving you."

— Exodus 20 (12)

As I write the preface for this book, my memory goes back twenty years when I joined the Centre for Development Studies to teach in the International Training Programme on Population and Development, a programme sponsored by the United Nations Fund for Population Activities, New York. I wrote my first article on ageing titled 'Aging in Kerala: One More Population Problem' in June 1989 for *Asia Pacific Population Journal*, an official organ of the United Nations Economic and Social Commission for Asia and Pacific (UNESCAP).

During the course of last twenty years, I have done projects for the Economic and Social Commission for Asia and Pacific, World Bank, HelpAge International, South Asian Network of Economic Institutes, Indo-Dutch Programme on Alternatives in Development, Shastri Indo-Canadian Institute and Canadian Institute of Health Research with various researchers in the field.

My first book was the one I co-authored with Dr U.S. Mishra and Dr P.S. Sarma. The book, titled *India's Elderly: Burden or Challenge?* was published in 1999 – the International Year of Elderly Persons. My second book was with Professor Phoebe S. Liebig, recipient of a Fulbright Senior Scholar Award, who had come to work on old-age homes and services in India. During our meeting, we decided to work on the proposal to edit a special issue of the *Journal of Aging and Social Policy* on India, published by the Haworth Press, USA. We brought out a special issue under the title, 'An Aging India: Perspectives, Prospects and Policies', Volume 15, Nos. 2 and 3. Later, the special issue was converted into a book, published by the Haworth Press, USA in 2003. Owing to its large demand in South Asia, the book was reprinted by Rawat Publications, Jaipur, in 2005.

During the last few years, most of my time has gone into developing a Research Unit on International Migration set up by the Ministry of Overseas Indian Affairs, Government of India, in 2006. However, I could consolidate and convert some of my earlier project reports into two books and publish them in 2008. The first one was titled *Social Security for the Elderly: Experiences from South Asia* based on my five-country studies in South Asia funded by the South Asian Network of Economic Institutes (SANEI). The second one titled *Institutional Provisions and Care for the Aged: Perspectives from Asia and Europe* was based on the project funded by the Indo-Dutch Programme on Alternatives in Development (IDPAD) that I had coordinated along with Myrtle Perera of Marga Institute, Sri Lanka and Professor Carla Risseeuw of the Department of Anthropology and Development Sociology, University of Leiden, Netherlands.

Though I met Dr Shanthi Johnson for the first time in Valencia Forum, Valencia, Spain, in April 2002, prior to the Second World Assembly on Ageing held in Madrid, Spain, from April 8 to 12, I was impressed by her work on ageing and nutrition. In 2003, when the Shastri Indo-Canadian Institute advertiezed for the Shastri Applied Research Project (SHARP) between researchers in Canada and India, Shanthi Johnson approached me to apply for a joint project on Promoting Healthy Ageing through Community Development in India. We were informed on June 20, 2003 by Ms. Janet Knowles, Project Director of Shastri Indo-Canadian Institute that our joint project has been recommended for funding with a total grant of Canadian $ 117,000. Out of this grant, the CDS received Canadian $ 25,283 for conducting research in Kerala. During the project, we felt the need to organize a seminar on the subject of healthy ageing, with participants comprising leading experts both from India and Canada, to consolidate the existing work on the subject. When we requested additional funds to conduct the seminar at Centre for Development Studies, Kerala, the SHARP project management committee approved a supplementary grant of Canadian $ 13,100 inclusive of the workshop cost $ 9,300.

At around the time when we were thinking about the seminar on healthy ageing in 2005, the Indian Academy of Geriatrics also proposed to organize their annual seminar under Dr D. Dalus from the Thiruvananthapuram Medical College. As a workshop coordinator of

'Healthy Ageing', I met him and we decided to organize both meetings together during December 2–4, 2005. Due to financial constraints, we invited experts mostly from India. This volume is mainly the outcome of this seminar. To fill the gap in the volume, we also requested few more authors to write papers. In total, out of 15 authors who contributed to the volume, 12 are from India and three from Canada. The seminar was organized at the Centre for Development Studies and it was attended by Dr K.N. Nair, Director; Dr M. Vijayanunni, IAS, Chief Secretary, Government of Kerala; Dr Rajan Khobragade, IAS, Additional Health Secretary, Government of Kerala; Ms. Sheela Thomas, IAS, Director, Census Operations; Mr Alok Sheel, IAS, Finance Resource Secretary, Government of Kerala and Ms. Lida Jacob, IAS, Secretary, Social Welfare, Government of Kerala alongwith all the authors of article included in the book except Mr Subratha Mukherjee and Mr Jean-Frederic Levesque. I am thankful to Dr K.N. Nair, Director, for all his help and support.

Dr S. Irudaya Rajan
Co-Investigator
SHARP Project on Promoting Healthy Ageing

1 Demographic Ageing, Nutrition and Disease Pattern in India

S. Irudaya Rajan and C. Shanthi Johnson

Population ageing is likely to become a prevailing element of social change around the globe. This establishes a number of serious challenges that range from social security coverage to increasing needs for health care, changing consumer behaviour, and possibly changes in productivity. An inevitable consequence of the demographic transition and the shift to lower fertility and mortality has been the evolution in the age structure. The current level and pace of population ageing vary widely by geographic region, and usually within regions as well, but virtually all nations are now experiencing growth in their numbers of elderly persons. Projected increases in both the absolute and relative size of the elderly population in many low and middle income countries is a subject of growing concern for public policy (Kinsella and Velkoff, 2001; World Bank, 2001; United Nations, 2002; Bordia and Bhardwaj, 2003; Liebig and Irudaya Rajan, 2003; Bose and Shankardass, 2004). The combination of high fertility and declining mortality during the twentieth century has resulted in large and rapid increases in the elderly population as successively larger cohorts step into old age, thus creating unprecedented increase of elderly persons in the twenty-first century. Since these demographic changes have been accompanied by rapid and profound socio-economic changes, cohorts might differ in their experience as they join the ranks of the elderly.

As of 2006, the number of persons aged 60 years or above in the world was estimated to be 600 million or 10 per cent of the total population. In terms of major regions, 53 per cent of the world elderly lives in Asia, while Europe has the next largest share with 24 per cent. The percentage of the elderly was much higher in the more developed regions (20%) compared to the less developed regions (8%), followed by the least developed countries (5%). Asia's share of the older population will increase to 63 per cent by 2050. Obviously, the two major population giants of Asia, namely, India (Irudaya Rajan, Mishra and Sarma 1999) and China will contribute a significant proportion to this growing elderly persons (Irudaya Rajan, Mishra and Sarma, 2003) and it will have long-lasting impact on social, economic and health status of the age structure in the next few decades.

According to the United Nations (2005) assessment, the number of people older than 60 years would triple between now and 2050, and their share of the total population would rise from 10.4 per cent to 21.7 per cent. Just 50 years ago, in 1950–55, global life expectancy at birth was about 47 years; by 2000–05, it had reached 65 years. Although life spans are longest in the industrial countries, people in developing countries are also living longer, with the average levels rising from 41 years in 1950–55 to 63 years in 2000–05, and projected to reach 74 years in 2045–50. In the typical sequence, the transition begins with successes in preventing infectious and parasitic diseases that benefit infants and young children most. Other things being equal, this initial decline in mortality generates a younger population age structure. After initial and sometimes very rapid gains in infant and child mortality have been achieved, further mortality declines increasingly benefit older ages and are eventually accompanied by fertility declines. Both changes contribute to reverse the early effect of mortality decline on the age structure. The process first started in low fertility western societies and then in Japan and now is spreading to the developing countries of Asia (United Nations, 2005).

Population Ageing Phenomenon in the Indian Context

The 2001 census has shown that the elderly population of India consisting of 28 states and seven Union Territories accounted for 77 million. It is interesting to note that the elderly constituted only 24 million in 1961; it increased to 43 million in 1981 and to 57 million in 1991. The proportion of elderly persons in the population of India rose from 5.63 per cent in 1961 to 6.58 per cent in 1991 (Irudaya Rajan, Mishra and Sarma, 1999) and to 7.5 per cent in 2001. This is also true of other older age cohorts. The elderly population aged 70 and above which was only 8 million in 1961 rose to hefty 21 million in 1991 and to 29 million in 2001. Besides, the proportion of the elderly above 70 in total population increased from 2.0 per cent in 1961 to 2.9 per cent in 2001. While in 1961, Indian population census reported 99,000 centenarians, their number rose to 138,000 in 2001. The growth rate among different cohorts of the elderly such as 60 plus, 70 plus and 80 plus during the decade 1991–2001 was much higher than the general population growth rate of 2 per cent per annum. However, the sex ratio among the elderly in India has favoured males as against the trend prevalent in other parts of the world (Table 1.1 and 1.2).

Table 1.1 ***Number and Proportion of the Elderly in the Indian Population by Age Groups, 1961–2001***

Age	*Number (in Millions)*					*Per cent of Elderly to the total population*				
	1961	1971	1981	1991	2001	1961	1971	1981	1991	2001
60+	25	33	43	57	77	5.6	6.0	6.49	6.76	7.5
70+	9	11	15	21	29	2.0	2.1	2.33	2.51	2.9
80+	2	3	4	6	8	0.6	0.6	0.62	0.76	0.8
90+	0.5	0.7	0.7	1	1.8	0.1	0.1	0.1	0.2	0.2
100+	0.01	0.01	0.01	0.01	0.1	0.02	0.02	0.02	0.02	0.01

Source: Irudaya Rajan, 2006.

Table 1.2 ***Sex Ratio and Growth Rate among the Indian Elderly, 1971–2001***

Age	*Sex Ratio of Elderly (males per 1,000 females)*				*Growth of Elderly (%)*		
	1971	1981	1991	2001	1971–81	1981–91	1991–2001
60+	1066	1042	1075	1028	2.78	2.72	3.04
70+	1030	1026	1084	991	3.13	3.08	3.32
80+	950	990	1090	1051	2.54	4.35	2.35
90+	897	892	1019	1131	0.66	5.08	n.a
100+	798	844	896	1782	0.19	0.44	n.a

Source: Irudaya Rajan, 2006.

India is one of the few countries in the world where males out number females. This phenomenon among the elderly is intriguing because female life expectancy at ages 60 and 70 is slightly higher than that of males. However, at any given age, contrary to what we would normally expect that there are more widows than widowers. Reasons for this unusual phenomenon need to be identified in a wider context. Since the beginning of the 20th century, life expectancy at birth among Indian males had been higher than that among females until the first half of the 1990s. Apart from this unusual demographic pattern of excess female mortality at infancy and childhood ages, the analysis is further complicated by the phenomenon of age exaggeration among the aged. Thus, the above observation of more males in old age does not reveal a true picture of the elderly persons (Irudaya Rajan, Mishra and Sarma, 2003). In India, the sex ratio of the aged as well as that of the old-old favours males. Reasons for more males in old age may consist of under-reporting of females, especially widows, age exaggeration, low female life expectancy at birth, and excess female mortality among infants, children and adults (Sudha and Irudaya Rajan 2003; Mari Bhat, 2002).

In addition, improvement in life expectancy at all ages will allow more old people to survive, thus intensifying the ageing process. In this context, an examination of the increasing life expectancy indicates that the gain will be shared by the older people and will increase their longevity. Table 1.3 provides evidence to support this. As can be seen, males are expected to live 16 years beyond age 60 and 10 years beyond age 70 and the corresponding years for females are 18 and 11 respectively. Urban females are expected to live for an additional two years at age 60 compared to their rural counterparts.

Table 1.3 ***Expectation of Life at Ages 60 and 70 for India***

Period	*Male*			*Female*		
	e^0	e^{60}	e^{70}	e^0	e^{60}	e^{70}
1970–75	50.5	13.4	8.6	49.0	14.3	9.2
1976–80	52.5	14.1	9.6	52.1	15.9	10.9
1981–85	55.4	14.6	9.7	55.7	16.4	11.0
1986–90	57.7	14.7	9.4	58.1	16.1	10.1
1991–95	59.7	15.3	10.0	60.9	17.1	11.0
1995–99	60.8	15.7	10.3	62.5	17.7	11.6
1996–00	61.0	15.8	10.4	62.7	17.8	11.7
1997–01	61.3	16.0	10.6	63.0	18.1	11.9

Source: Irudaya Rajan, 2006.

The assessment of India's demographic future, the age structure of the population was projected using the 2001 census age data published by the Registrar General of India as the base population; assumptions on future fertility and mortality trends are based on past trends as revealed by the Sample Registration System and other sources such as the first and second round of National Family Health Surveys (Visaria and Irudaya Rajan, 1999; Guilmoto and Irudaya Rajan, 2001) and our own understanding of the India's demographic regimes over the past 50 years (Irudaya Rajan and Aliyar, 2006). The projection period ranges from 2001 to 2051. It is also important to note that the number of projected elderly persons above 60 years of age in 2051 were already 10 years old in 2001. Given our assumptions regarding mortality, the projections are likely to be valid.

According to the population projections, the size of India's elderly population aged 60 and above is expected to increase from 77 million in 2001 to 179 million in 2031 and further to 301 million in 2051 (Table 1.4).

Table 1.4 ***Number, Proportion and Sex Ratio of the Elderly, 2001–2051***

	2001	2011	2021	2031	2041	2051
60 and above						
Numbers (in million)	77	96	133	179	236	301
Percentage to the total population	7.5	8.2	9.9	11.9	14.5	17.3
Sex Ratio (males per 1,000 females)	1,028	1,034	1,004	964	1,008	1,007
70 and above						
Numbers (in million)	29	36	51	73	98	132
Percentage to the total population	2.9	3.1	3.8	4.8	6.0	7.6
Sex ratio (males per 1,000 females)	991	966	970	930	891	954
80 and above						
Numbers (in million)	8	9	11	16	23	32
Percentage to the total population	0.5	0.7	0.8	1.0	1.4	1.8
Sex ratio (males per 1,000 females)	1,051	884	866	843	774	732

Note: According to the 2001 census, India was administratively divided into 28 states and 7 Union Territories.

Source: S. Irudaya Rajan and Sabu Aliyar. 2006.

The proportion is likely to reach 12 per cent in 2031 and 17 per cent in 2051. The number of elderly persons above 70 years of age (old-old) is likely to increase more sharply than those of 60 years and above. The old-old are projected to increase five-fold during 2001–2051; from 29 million to 132 million. Their proportion is expected to rise from 2.9 to 7.6 per cent. The oldest old (80+) among the elderly in India is expected to grow faster than any other age groups in the population. In absolute terms, it is likely to increase four-fold from 8 million in 2001 to 32 million in 2051. Figure 1.1 shows the percentage of elderly in the population by sex from 1901 to 2051.

Figure 1.1 ***Percentage of the Elderly 60 and Above by Sex, 1901–2051***

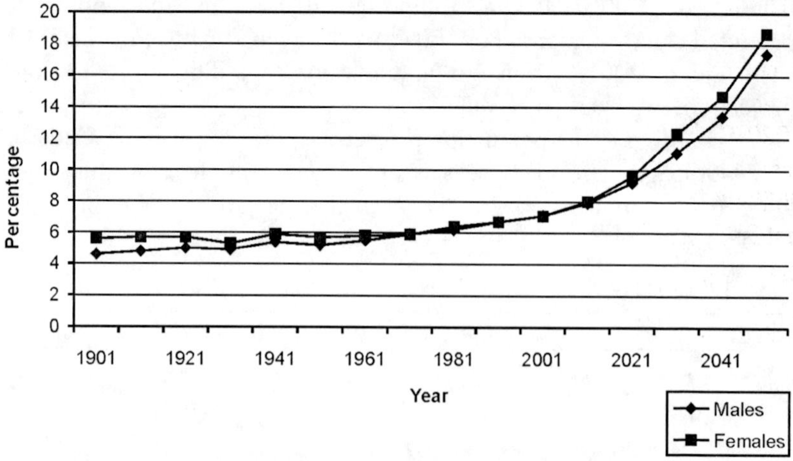

Reasons for Concern: The Challenges of being an Older Adult in India

According to World Health Organizations (WHO), "Longer life can be both a penalty and a prize". Population ageing, which is touted as humanity's greatest triumph, is also one of our greatest challenges. Prolongation of life span does not imply that the extra years bring continued health and prosperity. Ageing, marked by these aforementioned trends, is said to put an increased burden on the social, economic, and health care demands of all counties, especially in developing countries such as India (United Nations, 2002). The rapid population ageing will contribute to dramatic changes in the social fabric and in the structure of nations. Quality of life, level of familial support, and income generation are all major concerns of an ageing society. Demographic trends, such as the increasing number of the elderly, the decreasing number of children available to give support, and the stagnant economic infrastructure, coalesce to create further challenges to the ageing population that must be met with appropriate policy and action.

A challenge to ensuring the health and quality of life of the ageing population is the double burden of diseases and disability, especially in developing countries, which still struggle with infectious diseases and malnutrition as well as the recent, rapid growth of non-communicable diseases such as diabetes, cardiovascular diseases, and hypertension. In later years, non-communicable diseases (NCDs) become the main harbinger of death and disability. In 1998, NCDs were the cause of almost 60 per cent of deaths in the world, 77 per cent of those deaths occurred in developing countries (WHO, 2000). Statistical trends indicate that we can expect an increase in NCD deaths to 73 per cent in 2020. In addition, osteoporosis which is a debilitating bone disease associated with progressive decline in bone mass and increased susceptibility to fragility fracture is common among older individuals. In the last few years, the WHO and world health experts have been cautioning the impending osteoporosis epidemic in the developing world (Johnson, Irudaya Rajan and McLeod, 2003). Yet, in many developing countries including India, osteoporosis is not recognized as a source of concern.

Table 1.5 ***Distribution of Hospitalized Cases among per 1,000 Elderly Persons During the Last 365 days by Chronic Diseases, India, 2004***

Chronic Diseases	*Elderly*	*All ages*
Heart disease	109	54
Respiratory disorder	78	33
Diseases of urinary system/Renal disease	59	41
Diabetes mellitus	44	20
Hypertension	42	23
Neurological disorders	40	32
Disorder of joints and bones	34	25
Cancer and other tumours	30	29
Prostatic disorder	7	4

Note: Only conditions shown to be higher in elderly are reported.

Source: National Sample Survey Organisation (2006).

In the recent National Sample Survey Organisation (2006) data, highest distribution of hospitalized cases per 1,000 elderly persons was found for heart disease, respiratory disorders, renal diseases, hypertension, neurological disorders, joint and bone disorders and cancer compared to all ages as shown in Table 1.5. While these figures indicate that there is a higher distribution of hospitalization due to these chronic conditions, only a small fraction of those with these conditions are hospitalized. As such, the actual disease distributions are much higher than the hospitalization rates.

Also, based on the NSS (1995–96) data, one-fourth of the elderly in India have reported not suffering from any chronic disease. However, 75 per cent reported having at least one chronic disease. One out of two elderly persons in India suffers from at least one chronic disease which requires life-long medication. The proportion is slightly higher in urban areas (30%) compared to rural areas (20%). Not much difference has been observed between sexes. However, among the regions, north-west reported the highest proportion of the elderly with no disease, followed by west and south. The lowest proportion was reported by states in the east region. Similar patterns were observed among ages above 70 and also above 80.

Table 1.6 ***Disease Profile of the Elderly in India 1995–96***

Chronic Diseases	*Rural*			*Urban*			*Total*		
	Male	Female	Total	Male	Female	Total	Male	Female	Total
None	20.92	20.98	20.95	30.39	29.11	29.74	24.47	24.17	24.32
One	53.90	51.76	52.85	54.66	55.11	54.89	54.18	53.07	53.63
Two	20.15	19.43	19.80	21.87	23.08	22.48	20.80	20.86	20.83
Three or more	2.41	2.01	2.21	4.29	4.30	4.30	3.12	2.91	3.01

Note: Based on the raw data of NSS 1995–96.

Another layer of health concern is *disability* caused by age-related changes in physical health, including mobility and ability to perform activities of daily living (Manton, Stallard, and Corder, 1998). Five types of disabilities are usually reported in the ageing and health literature. They consist of visual impairment, hearing problem, difficulty in walking (locomotor problem), problems in speech and senility (Table 1.7). In India, 75 per cent of aged individuals are afflicted by at least one of these physical disabilities (National Sample Survey Organisation, 1998). Joint problems or mobility disability was reported in 72.4 per cent of the elderly (National Sample Survey Organisation, 1998). Darshan, Sharma and Singh (1987) reported that the major physical disability among the elderly in India consists of blindness and deafness. Shah (1993) in his study of urban elderly in Gujarat found deteriorating physical conditions among two-thirds of the elderly, consisting of poor vision, impairment of hearing, arthritis and loss of memory. The

1995–96 NSSO data showed that twenty five per cent of the elderly in India suffered from visual impairment, followed by hearing difficulties (14%) and locomotor disability and senility (each 11%). The prevalence rates of all the five disabilities were higher in rural than in urban areas. Except in respect of visual impairment, women were ahead in all the disabilities compared to males.

Table 1.7 ***Disabilities among the Elderly in India 1995–96***

Disabilities	*Rural*			*Urban*			*Total*		
	Male	Female	Total	Male	Female	Total	Male	Female	Total
Visual	27.12	26.71	26.92	24.46	25.22	24.85	26.39	26.32	26.36
Hearing	15.47	16.81	16.12	12.26	14.26	13.23	14.57	15.96	15.24
Speech	3.93	4.48	4.19	3.65	3.23	3.45	3.80	4.14	3.96
Locomotor	10.83	11.31	11.06	9.23	9.02	9.14	10.33	10.71	10.51
Amnesia/ Senility	10.13	10.92	10.51	7.67	8.36	8.02	9.36	10.13	9.73

Note: Based on the raw data of NSS 1995–96.

About 60 per cent of the elderly in India live disability-free lives in old age. The proportion of those with no disability was slightly higher among rural areas compared to urban areas. Among the five disabilities under investigation in the NSS survey, 40 per cent of the elderly reported suffering from at least one disability – slightly higher among females compared to males. Sex differentials were reported for the prevalence of two and three disabilities; 15 per cent suffered from at least two disabilities and another 6 per cent suffered from three disabilities in India. Most recent NSSO data showed that visual and mobility impairments are the most common among the elderly (NSSO, 2006).

Table 1.8 ***Disability Profile among the Elderly in India 1995–96***

Disability	*Rural*			*Urban*			*Total*		
	Male	Female	Total	Male	Female	Total	Male	Female	Total
None	59.33	57.45	58.41	63.41	61.87	62.63	60.86	59.18	60.03
One	39.30	40.69	39.98	35.03	36.62	35.83	37.70	39.09	38.39
Two	16.08	17.49	16.77	12.74	13.84	13.30	14.83	16.05	15.44
Three	6.38	6.84	6.61	4.59	4.82	4.70	5.71	6.05	5.88

Note: Based on the raw data of NSS 1995–96.

Besides chronic diseases and physical disabilities, psychiatric morbidity is also prevalent among a large proportion of the elderly. An enquiry in this direction by Gupta and Vohra (1987) provides evidence of psychiatric morbidity among the elderly. The physical health concerns are often compounded by increasing psychosocial problems, as the traditional extended family structure experiences breakdown and the elderly find themselves isolated and experiencing loneliness and depression. The mental and emotional challenges of ageing have yet to receive proper acknowledgement and support. Prakash (2001b) writes that, "Mental health issues receive little attention in India". The Mental Health Policy (MHP) of Kerala, states that "[it is a] common misconception that prevalence of mental illness is low in India particularly as compared to the West" (Praveenlal, Shaji and Mohandas, 1998). The MHP also recognises that Kerala lacks understanding of the mental health situation "because of lack of epidemiological data". Mental health is a significant health issue facility for the elderly population in India.

Table 1.9 ***Proportion (number per 1,000) of Aged Persons Who Cannot Move and are Confined to Bed or Home, India, 2004***

Age-group (years)	*Rural*			*Urban*		
	Male	Female	Total	Male	Female	Total
60–64	27	34	31	33	34	33
65–69	51	50	51	34	63	50
70–74	79	132	105	77	116	97
75–79	117	163	139	113	185	147
80 and above	220	326	269	239	323	283
All aged	67	88	77	68	100	84

Source: National Sample Survey Organisation (2006).

Chronic morbidity and physical impairments in the old age adversely affects mobility and capacity to perform personal self care and can confine the elderly to their home or bed (Arber and Ginn, 1991). Nearly 8 per cent of the elderly in India are immobile, while a disproportionately higher percentage of women are immobile compared to men (9.1% vs 6.8%). The results of NSSO (2006) reveal that the prevalence of immobility increases with the advance in age among the 60+ age group. The gender differences also intensify with the advance in age. Much evidence is available in health literature which suggests that women report more health problems despite their longevity across countries and cultures; moreover the gender differentials are particularly sharp for more severe limitations on physical functioning in the older age groups (Strauss et al., 1993). Further it was found that there is a slightly higher rate of immobility among the aged in the urban settings especially in the higher age groups. This could be due to a possible unfriendly or even adverse environment in the urban areas which could be hampering the mobility of aged persons with disabling conditions.

Disability and impairments leading to immobility among the elderly is a cause of concern for the ageing individuals as it adversely affects their quality of life increasing their risk of dependence and loss of autonomy. Meanwhile the society has to deal with difficult issues like increasing demands on social and medical care for such older persons. The average hospitalization rate in the country per 1,00,000 aged persons is 7,633. There is considerable gender difference in the rate of hospitalization as a much greater proportion of men are hospitalized as compared to their female counterparts (8,565 vs 6692 per 1,00,000). This is contrary to our expectation of higher health care utilization among older females based on our previous analysis which revealed a female disadvantage in terms of various health indicators. This indicates a gender bias in utilization of health care services. Similarly there is rural disadvantage in utilization of inpatient care services with only 6,636 rural aged persons being hospitalized as against 10,746 urban elderly per 1,00,000 elderly persons. The rural urban difference in the rate of hospitalization stems from the lack of availability of hospitals with inpatient care facilities in the rural areas. The diseases among the elderly for which there are more hospitalized cases than the rest are heart disease, cataract and bronchial asthma. Other common health problems requiring hospitalization are accidents/injuries/burns/fractures/poisoning, diseases of kidney/urinary system and diabetes mellitus. Among older women cataract tops the list of diseases requiring inpatient care followed by heart disease. While among older men heart disease followed by bronchial asthma has the highest reported cases of hospitalization. Similarly in the urban areas heart disease and cataract while in rural areas cataract and bronchial asthma have the highest rate of hospitalization.

The prevalence of disease and disability also reflects in the self-perceived health among the elderly. As a result of the double burden of diseases and increasing physical and psychosocial problems, only 6 per cent of the elderly reported "good health"; 69 per cent had "moderate health"; while 20 per cent had "poor health"; and 5 per cent had "very poor health" (Nayar, 2000).

Table 1.10 ***Self-Reported Current Health Status of the Elderly by Sex and Location, 2004***

Current state of health	*Rural*			*Urban*			*Total*		
	Male	Female	Total	Male	Female	Total	Male	Female	Total
Excellent	4.8	2.8	3.8	7.1	4.4	5.7	5.3	3.2	4.3
Good	65.0	62.1	63.6	69.1	68.2	68.6	66.1	63.9	65.0
Poor	26.6	31.3	28.9	21.6	24.9	23.3	25.3	29.5	27.4

Source: National Sample Survey Organisation (2006).

Self-assessed current health status is a subjective measure closely associated with the feelings of well-being and quality of life. In the survey when asked to rate their health status (as 'excellent', 'very good', 'good/fair' or 'poor'), nearly 70 per cent of the aged reported their health status to be ranging from 'excellent' to 'good/fair' while more than a quarter of the elderly reported their current health to be poor. Further it was found that a slightly higher per cent of the aged women report their health to be poor as compared to their male counterparts. In line with the previous research findings, more elderly persons from rural areas report health status as compared to those in urban areas. Significantly, it has been noted in the analysis of the previous rounds (NSS 52nd round) that such a high percentage of positive assessment of health status is despite a large number of the aged reporting to be suffering from at least one disability or chronic ailment (Sreerupa, 2006). It appears that quite a few of the aged persons are assessing their health based on a general perception which associates old age with illness and health problems. To better understand the association of self-reported health status with actual morbidity condition, the elderly respondent's perception about own health has been disaggregated on the basis of presence or absence of any ailment during the last 15 days prior to the interview in Table 1.11.

Table 1.11 reveals that more than 55 and 63 per cent of the elderly were reporting their health status to 'good/fair' despite suffering from some kind of ailment in rural and urban areas respectively. On the other hand, nearly 17 and 13 per cent of the elderly in rural and urban settings respectively were reporting poor health status although they have no ailments. Further, it is found that a higher percentage of rural as compared to the urban elderly persons perceive their health status to be poor both when they are sick and are not ailing. Apart from the rural urban difference in reporting there are gender differences in reporting of health status. It appears that more women report their health status to be poor when suffering from an ailment as compared to their male counterparts, while more men report good health status despite sickness. Similarly more elderly women, than men, report poor health status even when they report to be not suffering from any ailment in the last 15 days.

Table 1.11 ***Distribution of Aged Persons (per 1,000) by Own Perception About their Health, India, 2004***

Own perception about current state of health	*Aged persons with sickness*			*Aged persons without sickness*		
	Male	Female	Person	Male	Female	Person
				Rural		
Excellent	1.9	1.4	1.7	8.1	4.3	6.2
Good/Fair	58	52.5	55.3	77.2	77	77.1
Poor	40.1	46	42.9	14.7	18.7	16.7
				Urban		
Excellent	3.1	1.9	2.4	11.4	7.2	9.2
Good/Fair	64.1	62	63.1	77.5	78	77.8
Poor	32.7	36	34.5	11.1	14.8	13

Note: The proportions have been adjusted excluding the 'not reported cases'.

The first impression that we get from Table 1.11 is that the rural elderly and older women tend to be pessimistic about their health status where as the urban elderly as well as older men are more positive while assessing their health when the presence of an ailment in the lest 15 days is controlled. However, we need to take into consideration a few factors before interpreting the results. Apart from the obvious inference discussed above the difference in reporting could also be rooted in the poor utilization of health services among older women and the rural elderly. So when it comes to the reporting of ailments requiring formal diagnosis, it is quite possible that the female respondents may underreport (Sengupta and Agree, 2003). As a result although these elderly persons feel that their health status was poor they would not report any specific ailment. Meanwhile there have been studies which have found self-perceived health to be a reliable predictor of future functional status and even mortality (Idler and Benyamini 1997; Idler and Kasl, 1995). Hence there is a need for further research to have a closer look at the reasons for the differences in reporting health status.

Rising to the Challenge: The Importance of Health Promotion and Active Ageing

When considering the demographic inversion and associated challenges, it becomes evident that investments in ageing and health are necessary to ensure human rights and sustainable development. Given that people are living longer and the proportion of older adults in our society is higher, understanding the ageing process and facilitating healthy ageing is and will be critically important. Unless vigorous measures are taken to prevent non-communicable diseases commonly associated with the ageing process and to promote health during old age, the ageing of the population will place new and perhaps difficult demands on health care systems and younger generations. Meeting these challenges requires a clear understanding of the health needs of older adults, innovative planning to develop programmes, systems and structures which will support the health and welfare of the ageing population, and substantial reforms and policies at global, national, and local levels. Recently, the WHO's discussion paper on health and ageing indicated that "we can afford to get old if countries, regions and international organizations enact 'active ageing' policies and programmes that enhance the health, independence, and productivity of older women and men. The time to plan and to act is now". Active ageing is the process of optimizing opportunities for physical, social and mental well-being throughout the life course in order to extend healthy life expectancy, productivity and quality of life in old age. Active refers not only to physical activity but also to continuing involvement in social, economic, spiritual, cultural and civic affairs. Similar ideas have been conveyed in the 2002 International Strategy for Action on Aging. In addition to the call for awareness of ageing issues and challenges, WHO and the UN have issued policy framework and priority directions for action and research, which identify health and independence/ autonomy, productivity and protection of the ageing population as the three critical pillars essential for active ageing.

Active ageing promotes the level of health required for the elderly to continue as productive members of society, and saves them from the position of being mere recipients of care and services. In turn, this will benefit India's younger population who often take on the burden of caring for the elderly. Indeed, the country as a whole benefits from a healthy elderly population, a fact that high-income countries have recognized; they have been adjusting for some time to meet the needs of their older citizens. The governments of low-income countries are only just beginning to recognise the long-term socio-economic implications of their ageing populations. Health promotion has been shown to be effective in reducing the disease and disability burden.

In addition, there is a great need for suitable policies to promote active ageing in a coordinated and efficient manner. Currently, the well-being of older persons has been mandated in the Constitution of India. Specifically, the Article 41, which is a directive principle of the state policy, has it that the state shall make effective provisions for securing the rights to public assistance in care of old age. The National Policy on Older Persons visualises that the state shall extend support in the areas of: (i) financial security, (ii) health care, (iii) shelter, (iv) welfare, (v) protection against abuse and exploitation, and (vi) opportunities for the development of older person's potential. However, the actual translation of these policies into programme options is yet to materialize, particularly in the area of health promotion. Health care has been operating on the medical model of treating the diseases rather than preventing them through health promotion initiatives. In order to create efficient policies and programmes which will act in those areas exerting a negative influence on the health of the elderly, it is critical to understand the determinants of active ageing such as access to quality health care; health practices and beliefs of professionals, as well as of the elderly themselves; and the current health policies. Also, existing policies should be re-visited in the light of new and emerging trends.

As men and women live longer there will be an increase in aged persons with chronic illness and disability which is a matter of concern for the ageing individuals as well as the health care planners of the society. Chronic morbidities and disabling conditions adversely affect the quality of life of the elderly, increases their risk of financial dependence (Pal, 2004) and loss of autonomy. Meanwhile the society has to deal with difficult issues like increasing demands on social and medical care as well as growing cost of providing health care services to the chronically ill and disabled elderly. Thus, the health status of the aged should occupy an important place in any study of the elderly population. Ageing has become a global concern. As life expectancy increases so too does the need for information on improving the health of the growing elderly population.

Contribution of this Anthology: Overview of the Chapters

This anthology of collected articles seeks to promote healthy ageing, specifically in India. Covering a wide variety of topics it will serve as a reference book and will help to fill a gap in Indian resources available to practitioners and to the general public. Bringing together a formidable knowledge base, the collection will have two main thrusts. It will incorporate a great deal of medical knowledge on topics such as diabetes, arthritis, cardiovascular diseases, dementia and Alzhemer's, and mental health. It will also contain articles on lifestyle choices which foster good health, including nutrition, exercise and the prevention of abuse. Throughout the anthology there is a central focus: promoting healthy lifestyle choices through elderly-centred education and decision-making.

The first group of five articles, focus on specific disease preventions. The article entitled "Cardiovascular Health" maintains that vascular disease is so strongly age-related that it has been proposed as a biomarker of ageing. Dr Mathur explores the possible explanations for the dominant effect of age on the likelihood for occurrence of these cardiovascular diseases and the efficacies of different treatments. "Diabetes" looks at the epidemiology of the disease and the varying ways that it manifests itself. Dr Dalus recommends a multidimensional strategy which would put the "emphasis on prevention of diabetes and its complications," and he campaigns for an early intervention for vascular disease, and assessment of disability due to limb problems, eye disease, and stroke.

The article "Arthritis" explores the disease from diagnosis to treatment. Each component of the disease and its complicating factors are addressed. According to Dr Gambhir, "Arthritis (including Rheumatism) is one of the most common causes of loss of mobility, and confinement in bed or in house." The review article "Dementia and Alzheimer's disease" discusses the current status of prevalence, risk factors and management of the disease and its prevention. Dr Thakur takes us from symptoms through therapies and even to preventive lifestyle changes, always with an eye to minimizing the impact of the disease. In "Mental Health", Dr Kallivayalil describes mental health within the context of Indian mental health policies and other policies designed to support the elderly. He outlines where the policies are required and are not in place and where existing policies fall short of their mark. He highlights the ways in which the elderly people are at risk for depression and other mental health challenges. Dr Kallivayalil offers hope in the form of the information age. He sees great potential in the sharing of mental health knowledge and best practices globally.

The second group of five articles, focus on health promotion. The selected articles cover a range of issues often experienced by ageing people. The first article entitled "Health Promotion and Protection" presents the components of good health as defined by the WHO. Drs Krishnaswamy and Shanthi explore the multidimensional strategy needed to ensure well-being in old age. Health promotion is divided into two categories, one, to prevent and treat disease, and two, to screen for sub-clinical disease conditions with a goal of eradicating or at least limiting the chance and occurrence for disease.

In the article "Physical Activity and Ageing" Drs Jones and Johnson describe the benefits of physical activity as a means of mitigating the potential burden of an ageing population, through not only disease prevention, but even more importantly, through the preservation of physiological reserve capacity or fitness. Continued physical activity allows older adults to continue to perform many of the tasks of daily living required for independent function.

"Nutrition and Healthy Policy" and "Nutrition for Healthy" focus on the enormous role that foods play in promoting good health. In the first of the two articles Dr Natarajan deals with the increased needs for specific vitamins as the body ages. He describes a study, which he recently undertook, in the rural Indian community of Melmaruvathur. He demonstrates how a large percentage of the elderly Indian population is undernourished. The second nutrition article by Dr Puri focuses on the ways in which nutrition can help to compress "morbidity into a lesser time frame", allowing elderly people an opportunity to life free of disease for a longer period of time. Both nutrition articles promote healthier choices by sharing a wealth of information on diet.

The final of the second group of articles by Dr Shankardass entitled "Elder Abuse and Adult Protection" reports on "the lack of serious academic enquiry" into this major health concern. Faced with a dearth of governmental statistics, she has explored the various sociological avenues open to her, including news reports and small qualitative studies. Her article challenges the sectors of health and criminal justice to become involved in first seeing and then preventing abuse.

These articles seek to inform the public and the practitioners on a variety of topics related to ageing, with the ultimate aim of promoting good health for elderly people. The collection has articles from practitioners in the various fields, as well as from academics. All of the contributors are connected in some way with India. And all have evinced a respect for the people they seek to teach. The articles are readable and concise. Both in terms of plain language and well-defined ideas, and in terms of format this anthology will be accessible to medical personnel and to the general public alike.

References

Bordia, Anand and Gautam Bhardwaj (eds.), 2003. *Rethinking Pension Provision for India*. Tata Mcgraw-Hill Publishing Company Limited, New Delhi.

Bose, Ashish and Mala Kapur Shankardass. 2004. *Growing Old in India: Voices Reveal and Statistics Speak*. B.R. Publishing Corporation, New Delhi.

Guilmoto, Christophe Z. and S. Irudaya Rajan. 2001. "Spatial Patterns of Fertility Transition in Indian Districts". *Population and Development Review*, Vol. 27, No. 4, pp. 713–738.

Gupta, Punam and Adarsh K. Vohra. 1987. "Pattern of Psychiatric Morbidity in the Aged", in M.L. Sharma and T.M. Dak (eds.), *Aging in India*. Ajanta Publications (India), New Delhi, pp. 214–21.

Idler, E.L. and Y. Benyamini. 1997. "Self-rated Health and Mortality: A Review of Twenty Seven Community Studies". *Journal of Health and Social Behavior*, Vol. 38, No. 1, pp. 21–37.

Idler, E.L. and S.V. Kasl. 1995. "Self-ratings of Health: Do They Also Predict Change in Functional Ability?" *Journals of Gerontology: Social Sciences*, 50B: S344–S353.

Irudaya Rajan, S., U.S. Mishra and P.S. Sarma. 1999. *India's Elderly: Burden or Challenge?* Sage Publications, New Delhi and Thousand Oaks, London.

——. 2003. "Demography of Indian Ageing, 2001–2051". *Journal of Aging and Social Policy*, 15 (2 and 3), pp. 11–30.

Irudaya Rajan, S. 2006. "Chronic Poverty among Indian Elderly", in Asha Kapur Mehta and Andrew Sheperd (eds.), *Chronic Poverty and Development Policy in India*. Sage Publications, New Delhi, pp. 168–196.

Irudaya Rajan, S. and Sabu Aliyar. 2006. "Population Projections for India, 2001–2051". Chapter 1 in S. Irudaya Rajan, Carla Risseeuw and Myrtle Perera. *Care of the Aged*. IDPAD project report. Centre for Development Studies, Thiruvananthapuram, Kerala.

Johnson, C.S., S. Irudaya Rajan and W. McLeod. 2003. "Importance of Osteoporosis for the Aging Society in India: Status Review and Recommendations". *Indian Journal of Gerontology*: 17.

Kinsella, Kevin and Victoria A. Velkoff. 2001. "An Aging World: 2001". U.S. Census Bureau Series, P 95/01, Government Printing Office, Washington D.C.

Liebig, Phoebe and S. Irudaya Rajan (eds.), 2003. *An Aging India: Perspectives, Prospects and Policies*. The Haworth Press, New York.

Manton, K.G., E. Stallard and L.S. Corder. 1982. "The Dynamics of Dimensions of Age-related Disability 1982 to 1994 in the U.S. Elderly Population". *Journal of Gerontology: A Biological Science and Medical Science,* 1998, 53: B59–70.

Mari Bhat, P.N. 2002. "Maternal Mortality in India: An Update". *Studies in Family Planning,* 33 (3), pp. 227–236.

National Sample Survey Organisation. 1998. The Aged in India: A Socio-Economic Profile. NSS 52nd Round (July 1995–June 1996), Department of Statistics, Government of India.

——. 2006. "Morbidity, Health Care and the Condition of the Aged". NSS 60th Round (January–June 2004), Report No. 507, Ministry of Statistics and Programme Implementation, Government of India.

Nayar, P.K.B. 2000. "The Aging Scenario in Kerala: A Holistic Perspective". HelpAge India, 6: pp. 5–13.

Pal, S. 2004. "Do Children Act as Old Age Security in Rural India? Evidences from an Analysis of Elderly Living Arrangements". http://129.3.20.41/eps/lab/papers/0495/0405002.pdf

Prakash, I.J. 2001b. "New Hope in the New Millennium: Reasons for Optimism about Aging in the Future". HelpAge India, 7: pp. 1–6.

Praveenlal, K., K.S. Shaji and E.M. Mohandas. 1998. "Mental Health Policy for Kerala State: A Proposal from IPS Kerala State Branch" (10th October 1998), IPS Kerala.

Sengupta, M. and E.M. Agree. 2003. "Gender, Health, Marriage and Mobility Difficulty among Older Adults in India". *Asia-Pacific Population Journal*, Vol. 18, No. 4, December, pp. 53–65.

Shah, V.P. 1993. "The Elderly in Gujarat". Department of Sociology, Gujarat University, Ahmedabad (Mimeographed).

Sreerupa. 2006. "Gender, Ageing and Widowhood: Health Vulnerability and Socio-Economic Influences", Unpublished M.Phil. Dissertation, Centre for Development Studies, Thiruvananthapuram.

Strauss, J., P.J. Gertler, M.O. Rahman and K. Fox. 1993. "Gender and Life-Cycle Differentials in the Patterns and Determinants of Adult Health". *The Journal of Human Resources*, Vol. 28, No. 4, Special Issue:

Symposium on Investments in Women's Human Capital and Development, pp. 791–837.

Sudha, S. and S. Irudaya Rajan. 2003. "Persistent Daughter Disadvantage: Do Estimated Sex Ratio at Birth and Sex Ratios of Child Mortality Risk Reveal?" *Economic and Political Weekly*, 38 (41), October 11–17, pp. 4351–4360.

United Nations. 2002. "World Population Ageing, 1950–2050". Department of Economic and Social Affairs, Population Division, New York.

United Nations. 2005. World Population Prospects: The 2004 Revision. Department of Economics and Social Affairs, Population Division, New York.

Visaria, Pravin and S. Irudaya Rajan. 1999. "National Family Health Survey: A Landmark in Indian Surveys". *Economic and Political Weekly*, Vol. XXXIV, Nos. 42 and 43, pp. 3002–07.

World Bank. 2001. India: The Challenge of Old Age Income Security. Finance and Private Sector Development, South Asia Region, Report No. 22034–IN, Washington D.C.

World Health Organization. 2000. Non-communicable Disease Prevention and Health Promotion. Retrieved June 2003 from http://www.who.int/hpr/index.shtml.

2 Ageing and Well-being

A.B. Dey

Our perception of old age has not changed much since the time of Buddha when the glimpse of an aged person made Prince Siddhartha renounce the world some 2,500 years back. In the modern-day socio-economic context, being old often means to be ill, non-productive, poor, weak, demented, unattractive, dependent and abused. In such a situation, it is no surprise that most people view old age with apprehension and trepidation. Though, there would be many who enjoy the twilight years of life in health and vitality, it is a fact that older people in most communities have a large burden of ill-health and disability arising out of age-related decline of organ systems.

There are significant individual differences in every aspect of life in old age. Those who have lived through their childhood, youth and adult life in trying circumstances grow old in poor health and functionality with major shortcomings in social, economic and behavioural aspects of their lives. On the other hand, there are those who have lived well throughout their lives, have a positive ageing experience though some degree of age associated decline sets in. We all aspire to age healthily, with our mental faculties intact, rid of degenerative diseases and pain, and a brief terminal event to extinguish the flame of life.

"Normal/usual ageing" involves the degeneration of the physical structure and functions of organs, disease and disability. This is the state that everyone abhors and is apprehensive of. The state of health in old age depends on one's genetic endowment, the surrounding environment and the kind of lifestyle that one has lived during childhood and adulthood. The question is, can one alter one's susceptibility to disease and disability with the help of interventions? Though not much evidence is available to support this hypothesis, many of the health problems of old age are known to result from an unhealthy lifestyle and are therefore potentially preventable.

Long-term studies in developed societies have indicated that avoidance of smoking, not adopting a sedentary lifestyle and freedom from obesity can go a long way in preventing ill-health and inducing prosperity in the later years of life. However, in poor resource settings such as India, where most people slog throughout their lifetime for a mere day-to-day existence, exhaustion and malnutrition prove to be more powerful determinants of ill-health in the later part of life. The ultimate goal of all development is to prolong human life and make it pleasurable. Once that is achieved, longevity poses its own challenges that need innovative interventions never conceived before. Thus, there is a need to achieve "successful ageing" – a concept in which old age with all its disadvantages is still worth living. The only alternative to ageing is dying, and nobody wants to die young. In this essay an attempt will be made to quantify the diseases and declines of old age among older Indians and also to look at ways and means of ameliorating them.

Burden of Ill-Health and Disability

The increasing number of older people in Indian society has been well perceived from census data and has been dealt with elsewhere. The population over the age of sixty years has nearly tripled in last 50 years and the relentless increase continues in projected population figures by demographic experts. While population ageing is a success story of socio-economic development and good public health practice, it also denotes economic crisis, social crisis due to increased demand and inequitable supply; and progressive deterioration of health and functional status for individual leading to increase demand for services from various institutions of the civil society.

It is generally considered rather simplistically that health problems in old age are a cluster of problems such as increased susceptibility to infection, inability to cope with physical and psychological stress, degenerative arthritis, atherosclerotic and vascular diseases of heart and brain, cancer of various organs and cognitive impairment due to declining brain size or more importantly various types of dementing disorders. However, data from focused academic research as well as three nationwide sample surveys of 1986–1987, 1995–1996 and 2004 reveal that the magnitude and nature of diseases and disabilities of old age may be much more in magnitude than what has been summarized in the previous statement.

A landmark survey was conducted between 1984 and 1986 by Dr A. Venkoba Rao, Professor of Psychiatry, Madurai Medical College, Madurai, Tamil Nadu to determine the health problems in the rural elderly and health services available to them. This was the first Task Force project conducted by Indian Council of Medical Research (ICMR) on old age health. The study was carried out from the Kallandiri PHC in Madurai district through a geriatric clinic approach. 1910 subjects (males: 664 and females: 1246) were assessed in a cross sectional observation. The population studied was a reflection of typical rural Indian population with 91 per cent in socio-economic class IV and V (indicating poverty); a literacy rate of only 20 per cent and the death rate of 57 per thousand per annum. This socio-demographic description will probably hold true for many parts of India twenty years later today. The health problems in this population as detected by the primary care physicians included two important conditions, namely cataract related visual impairment and locomotor disability due to degenerative arthritis. It may be noted here that at that point of time, the National Blindness Control Programme targeting cataract related blindness was in its early phases. Nearly 90 per cent of this rural older population had cataract related blindness. Forty per cent of this group had locomotor disability indicating the need for assistance in activities of daily living. Other health problems arising out of diseases of major organ systems such as the brain and the nervous system, heart, lungs, gastrointestinal and genitourinary tract etc. were detected in reasonably high proportion of older subjects. Depression and other mental health problems were also detected in a tenth of the subjects. This study also detected acceptance of primary health care services among older subjects. Over the years, however, the level of satisfaction among older people regarding the PHC services have declined, which has necessitated affirmative action in strengthening of the primary health care services as a policy initiative on the part of the government.

There have been three nationwide sample surveys in last two decades to assess the socio-economic and health status of older Indians in 1986–87 (NSSO Survey 42nd round), 1995–96 (NSSO Survey 52nd round) and 2004 (NSSO Survey 60th round). The 42nd round of sample survey estimated about the prevalence of chronic disease at 45 per cent, and immobility at 5 per cent. The common problems were joint pain, high or low blood pressure, heart disease, cough, piles and visual impairment. The similarity of findings in the ICMR Task Force study in Madurai and 42nd round of sample survey were remarkable and were also not unexpected as both were conducted at a same time period. The 52nd round of sample survey reported a slightly higher prevalence of chronic disease at 52–55 per cent and the problems were nearly same as the 42nd round. The prevalence of disabilities were also assessed in this survey and were reported at about 40 per cent; visual impairment and hearing deficit being the most frequent, 25–27 per cent and 12–14 per cent, respectively. The prevalence of amnesia (possibly a surrogate question for cognitive impairment) was estimated at an alarming figure of 7–10.5 per cent (urban and rural figures respectively).

The latest round of survey (60th) reported that about 8 per cent of older Indians were confined to their home or bed; the proportion of such immobile or home bound people rose with age to 27 per cent after the age of 80 years and women were more frequently affected than males in both villages and cities. The 60th round of sample survey estimated the state of self-perceived health status of older people. A good or fair condition of health was reported by 55–63 per cent of people with a sickness and 77–78 per cent of people without one. In contrast about 13–17 per cent of survey population without any sickness reported ill-health. It is possible that many older people take ill-health in their stride as a part of "usual/normal ageing". This observation has a lot of significance as self-perceived health status is an important indicator of health service utilization and compliance to treatment interventions.

In a systematic review of all relevant research projects funded by ICMR, prevalence figures of three important diseases, namely, hypertension, diabetes and ischemic heart disease, were estimated and published in a landmark paper in the *Indian Journal of Medical Research* 1997. The prevalence of hypertension was 110 per thousand (males – 84 and females – 148) among rural people while it was 209 per thousand (males – 202 and females – 214) among urban people. The estimates for ischemic heart disease were: rural: 118/1,000 (males – 103 and females – 143) and urban: 234/1,000 (males – 228 and females – 241); and diabetes were: rural: 53/1,000 (males – 57 and females – 48) and urban: 165/1,000 (males – 166 and females – 154). The prevalence of two common disabilities was also studied, namely visual and hearing impairment. The prevalence of visual impairment was 172/1,000 (males – 135 and females – 224) in rural India and 141/1,000 (males – 99 and females – 192) in urban India. The prevalence of hearing impairment was estimated at 597/1,000 in rural areas where as it was 613/1000 in urban India. The authors made projections of number of patients in each of these diseases and disabilities for the year 1996. It was projected that out of a possible 63 million older people in India in the year 1996; there were 11 million older people with visual impairment; 38 million with hearing impairment, 9 million each with hypertension and ischemic heart disease, and 5 million with diabetes. These data only provide some glimpses of the burden of ill-health and disability older people carry and by no means provide the total picture. It is worth noting hear that there are many other health and functionality issue which have not yet been adequately addressed scientifically.

There have been some published reports on morbidity patterns in old age. A publication from South India provides the profile of diseases and symptoms reported by the older people from an urban location. The common diagnoses in this population were: anaemia 46.7 per cent, hypertension 31.8 per cent, diabetes 9.7 per cent, chronic obstructive pulmonary disease 9 per cent, IHD 2.4 per cent, stroke 1.7 per cent and thyroid disease 1.4 per cent. In the same population the common complaints were: joint pain 82.2 per cent, loss of memory 47 per cent, chest pain 38.1 per cent, lack of sleep 32.9 per cent, head ache 26.6 per cent, palpitation 22.5 per cent and cough 19.4 per cent. The data indicates lack of concordance between perceived health problems and the actual diagnosis arrived at in most instances. It is matter of debate therefore that whether a medical model of old age health issues (labelling names to lack of well-being) can really address the ground realities.

In another publication from North India, the disease and disability data from a Geriatric clinic was published. The report indicated that older people have limited number of common diseases to account for most of their illnesses. The ten most common diagnoses in this clinic were hypertension (39.5%), cataract (35.3%), osteoarthritis (33.7%), COPD (20%), IHD/CAD (19%), prostate enlargement in men (16%), diabetes (15.2%), dyspepsia (11%), constipation (irritable bowel syndrome) (9.2%) and depression (8.5%) which accounted for 81 per cent of all diagnoses while 95 per cent of all diagnoses were accounted for by 20 common problem in a dedicated facility in a tertiary care centre. Most people had multiple diagnoses; two diseases were diagnosed in 29 per cent, three in 25 per cent and four in 15 per cent of older patients in this facility. In addition 87 per cent of patients had one acute health problem or the other in the preceding one month. The report also noted physical dependence, stroke, osteoporosis, fragility fractures, heart failure, dementia as the common health problems for the very old people. In addition to the diseases mentioned above, several disabilities were also detected in the clinic population. These included: impaired vision (48.5%), impaired hearing (32%), inability to pursue activities of daily living (7%), impaired arm function (6.5%) impaired leg function (5%), cognitive impairment (5%), depressed mood (20%) urinary incontinence (20% largely in women). The observations of this paper can be summarized as multiple diseases (from common conditions), multiple disabilities and frequent acute health problems as the hallmark of old age health.

The mortality data of older people in India is sketchy and may not provide a clear picture of the actual causes of death. In rural India pneumonia and bronchitis account for 27 per cent of all deaths in old age while IHD (12.5%), stroke (9.8%), tuberculosis (7%) and cancer (5.8%) are the other common causes of death. Whereas in urban India cardiovascular disease (IHD and stroke included) account for 39 per cent of deaths in old age, while infection (13%), lung diseases (COPD and cancer – 10%), cancer (7%) ill-defined conditions account for 27 per cent of all deaths. However, as indicated, earlier accurate collection of data with clear definition of each diagnoses as a cause of death is required for a better understanding of the issue.

Research on old age health has not been very strong in India due to various reasons in the past. Most work has been done from a few centres. However, in recent years, many more reports on old age heath have been noticed after the Indian Academy of Geriatrics started publishing its own journal on a quarterly basis. It is expected that in coming years many more academicians and researchers will start publishing on various hitherto neglected and ignored issues in old age health in India.

Functionality and Disability of Ageing

In the preceding paragraphs an attempt has been made to provide a clinical account of health issues in old age. References to discordance between perceived health status and actual state of health among older people have also been made. Such discordance creates major difficulties for researchers and academicians in making a correct assessment of the challenge. Further, there may be over- or under-estimation of the burden of ill-health and disability in old age, which is likely prove to be a nightmare for the planner and policy maker. To overcome such difficulties, a functionality-disability approach may be adopted in describing the health status of older people, and it may provide a realistic account of the situation.

The physiological deterioration which sets in after post-maturational and post-reproductive phase distinguishes an older person from a younger one. Such physiological deterioration possibly determines the magnitude and impact of age associated morbidity and disability. This process of decline is by no means homogenous and steady in different individuals of same age, gender, social class, race, community and family. That is why, we begin to become dissimilar and heterogeneous as we age. The rate of functional decline is extremely variable even within the organs of the same individual. The decline in functionality is the result of damages in the organs and tissues that are not adequately repaired resulting in accumulation of defects in the entire system. The reasons for age-associated decline are: the intrinsic living process, extrinsic environmental and lifestyle factors, and diseases.

Damages Resulting from Intrinsic Living Process

Probably there is no activity in our life process that does not damage to organs. For example, aerobic metabolism which is essential for generation of metabolic energy from food, produces highly reactive compounds such as superoxide radicals, hydroxyl radicals and hydrogen peroxide. All these molecules cause oxidative damage to vital organs. Similarly, metabolism of the glucose, apart from providing energy, can lead to glycation of proteins and nucleic acids adversely affecting their function.

Damages Caused by Extrinsic Factors

The best example of the extrinsic factor that is associated with ageing is diet and calorie consumption in animal experiments. A broad range of physiological functions such as that of immune system and cardiovascular system; reproduction, gene expression etc. are maintained in a youthful state in calorie-restricted animals. The reverse phenomenon is also true in overfed and obese animals. Possibly human beings also behave in a similar manner. Lifestyle factors such as sedentary habits and physical exercise influence the ageing process in a contradictory manner. Other factors which may influence the ageing process are: occupation, environmental exposure and smoking. Though not extensively investigated, there is evidence to suggest that several psychosocial factors also affect the functional state in old age. These include: economic status, living arrangement, social network, emotional support and educational status.

Damage Resulting from Age-Associated Diseases

The age-associated diseases needs to be differentiated from the normal ageing process. It is generally accepted that a substantial degree of physiological deterioration in old age results from age-associated diseases. As many older people have one or more age-associated diseases, some degree of functional impairment is generally expected in a large majority of older persons.

Age-Associated Changes in the Functioning of Different Organ Systems

All organ systems demonstrate age-associated physiological deterioration. These changes have their origin at the molecular, receptor or cellular level. Denaturation of lens protein, poor responsiveness of β-adrenergic receptor and fall in creatinine clearance are some of the manifestations of the age-associated physiological decline. The net result of these changes are: decline in the ability to cope with challenges, decline in aerobic capacity, inability to maintain acid base homeostasis, decrease in lean body mass, increase in fat mass, fall in bone mass, inability to maintain body temperature and derangements in glucose homeostasis.

Physical Fitness

The functionality and physical fitness of an individual depend on one's state of health which includes physical, emotional, social and spiritual state. The determinants of health and fitness in old age are genetic endowment, environmental influences and lifestyle during adulthood. Though ageing of the human species begins immediately after conception, the physical decline becomes apparent only after the third decade of life, which marks the beginning of the post-reproductive phase. The level of physical fitness which determines the capacity of an individual to work, depends on four major features: cardiovascular stamina, muscle strength and power, flexibility, and psychomotor skill. All these skills decline with age. In addition, intactness of the major sensory input of vision and hearing, cognitive and affective mental health, nutritional status, ability to perform activities of daily living, continence, socio-economic status, safety of surrounding environment and availability of social and emotional support also have direct or indirect influence on an individual's physical fitness and functionality.

Frailty and Dependence

In contrast to fitness frailty is a state of health where the older person is dependent on others, experiencing loss of physiological reserves, having many chronic illnesses, having complex medical and psychosocial problems, experiencing uncoupling from the environment, being at a substantial risk of adverse health outcomes, having atypical disease presentations and simply experiencing accelerated ageing. The clinical characteristics of frailty are muscle weakness, fatigue, inactivity, slow and/or unsteady gait, weight loss, reduced endurance and impaired cognition. There are several biological correlates of frailty which range from abnormalities in hormone production to cytokine production and from sarcopenia to osteopenia.

There are several disease conditions which are responsible for frailty of old age. A detailed description of all of them will be beyond the scope of the article. An attempt will be made to give short narratives of issues related to cardiovascular health, bone heath and mental health for a clear perspectives of challenges of old age care.

Cardiovascular Health

Vascular diseases of heart and brain generate enormous amount of fear and interest in our mind irrespective of educational status and level awareness. This is invariably due to the risk of sudden death associated acute myocardial infarction or heart attacks in common language. Similarly every body dreads the possibility of a stroke or cerebro-vascular accident (a condition of the brain similar to heart attack) which may lead to death and even worse severe disability due to paralysis of the body.

Equally true is the fact that in the last quarter of the last century, there has been significant improvement in the outcome of acute myocardial infarction and stroke has improved substantially with thrombolytic therapy, primary percutaneous coronary interventions (angioplasty) with or without placement of stents inside coronary artery and even coronary artery bypass surgery. Failure of cardiac function which was earlier considered as incurable is now managed with cardiac transplant. While technology has improved the outlook of many serious and life threatening disorders, prevention of these conditions remains a challenge for the public health system.

There are two very common but potentially preventable heart disease in old age: ischaemic heart disease including acute myocardial infarction and heart failure. For the brain and the nervous system the conditions are stroke due to occlusion of cerebral blood vessels or bleeding into the brain substance and recurrent ischemic insult to the brain leading to the development of vascular dementia. It is now known from research in last fifty years that high blood pressure, high blood cholesterol and smoking are the primary reversible causes of these diseases in addition to non-modifiable factors such as race, gender, advancing age and family history.

Cardiovascular diseases including stroke constitute the most common cause of death in advancing years in most societies. Consequently prevention programmes involving smoking cessation, cholesterol and blood pressure control and reduction of obesity by diet control and physical activity have been adopted and advocated by most international and national health organizations. The effect of such programmes in developed societies are already discernible and needs to be promoted globally as a major initiative for health ageing.

Bone Health and Osteoporosis

Osteoporosis, a very common health problem in ageing women, is "a skeletal disorder characterized by compromised bone strength predisposing a person to an increased risk of fracture. Bone strength reflects the integration of two main features: bone density and bone quality." The clinically applicable index of bone quality for all practical purposes, according to the present state of knowledge, is a history of a fragility fracture provided by the patient. Clinically, a fragility fracture can be defined as one that occurs as a result of minimal trauma, such as a fall from a standing height or less, or no identifiable trauma. In the absence of any reliable methods of measuring bone quality, the diagnosis of osteoporosis tends is currently based on demonstration of low bone mineral density (BMD) by bone densitometry. The interpretation of BMD results have been standardized by WHO study group's definitions, which are based on a comparison of a patient's BMD with the mean for a normal young adult population of the same sex and race. The WHO criteria are derived from Caucasian postmenopausal women population and are, thus, best applicable to that group. However, in the absence of normative data from other races, WHO criteria have been widely accepted and used in clinical practice. Normative data for Indians are not available. It is possible that if we use the WHO criteria substantial number of patients may be over diagnosed and over treated. Thus it is imperative that normative data for major ethnic groups (such as Indians) be established or alternative methods for measurement of bone mass be developed. Indian literature has always focused more on male osteoporosis compared to osteoporosis in women. Reports published in 1960s and later in 1980s–1990s from hospitals indicate that hip fractures in males due to osteoporosis may be an important health problem in India. With the disadvantage of not having large scale studies, the clinical experience and extrapolated studies suggest that: (a) osteoporosis is not uncommon in India; (b) osteoporotic fractures (especially of hip) occur more commonly in Indian males than females; and (c) osteoporotic fractures usually occur 10–20 years earlier in Indian men and women, compared to Caucasian population. Though there are no authentic epidemiologic data on osteoporosis in India most conservative estimates India has nearly 30 million women with osteoporosis. (*Source*: Action Plan Osteoporosis, Osteoporosis Society of India).

Despite osteoporosis being recognized as an important health issue for the ageing population, the significance of this 'silent epidemic' has not yet been fully realized by policy makers and planners. Consequently, interventions for primary prevention of osteoporosis, prevention of first fracture, early detection and effective treatment have not yet been seriously implemented. Improvement of bone health in youth through calcium and vitamin supplementation, physical activity, early diagnosis by bone densitometry and treatment with recently evolving treatment strategy can substantially reduce the morbidity associated with this physiological change of skeletal system.

Mental Health in Old Age

There are several stresses of old age. These include (a) disruption of the family support system, (b) decrease in the economic status and independence, (c) challenges of living alone, (d) loneliness and consequent emotional problems, (e) challenges of adjustment, (f) physical and psychiatric morbidity, (g) widowhood exposing women to more physical and psychosocial risks, and (h) poor utilization of health and welfare services by older people. Beyond these stressful living conditions, older people have substantial mental health disorders, among them depression and dementia are the most important.

The prevalence rates of mental disorders in old age point towards a large burden of morbidity. Surveys have indicated rates of 89/1000 among people above 60 years. The range of mental morbidity which older people suffer from is the same as younger adults. Two very common disorders are unlikely to be picked up in epidemiological surveys, namely, anxiety disorders and acute confessional disorders or delirium. An elderly person may have beginning of anxiety symptoms as a result of a life-threatening physical illness. Delirium is usually the result of infections, heart failure, or very often medications. All such cases are likely to be missed in epidemiological surveys as they are short-lived, or are masked by the primary physical morbidity.

Depression

Depressive disorders are extremely common in old age, though they are is more likely to be missed or ignored by the clinicians as well as the general public. Various studies have reported that 10–15 per cent of elderly population suffer from significant and treatable depression. However, only a small proportion of depressed elderly seek help. Inadequate management increases the risks of morbidity and mortality in this age group. Till recently it was erroneously believed that older depressive patients had a uniformly bad prognosis. However, it is confirmed now that prognosis for elderly depressives is far from gloomy. Currently available tricyclic drugs (imipramine, nor-triptyline) and selective serotinine reuptake inhibitors (fluoxetine, sertraline, venlafaxine) all work very well in these cases. Most patients are helped by using these well-tried drugs when used in adequate doses and duration. ECT is also a safe and viable option. Death rate of these patients is consistently higher than expected when compared with general population, the reasons for which are not very clear.

Dementia

Dementia is a syndrome, produced by dysfunction of acquired of intellectual functions and neuropsychological activity. The syndrome occurs with a wide variety of conditions including degenerative, vascular, demyelinating, traumatic, neoplastic, hydrocephalic, inflammatory, infections, toxic and metabolic.

The likelihood of developing dementia increases with age. The most widely quoted estimates are that of 1 per cent of people at the age of 60 years, doubling every five years to about 30 per cent above 80 years experience cognitive impairment of sufficient severity to warrant the diagnosis of dementia. Reports from India suggest a prevalence of 2.7–3.6 per cent of older people as suffering from dementia.

An elderly population cannot be simply divided into cases of dementia and normal people. The distribution of cognitive decline runs on a continuum. Most cases who present themselves for clinical services are already into advanced stages of dementia. Those who are in the community with various degrees of cognitive decline, manifest social and behavioural changes mediated by personality and environmental factors. Memory impairment may be profound and yet a person may survive in the community if social behavioural skills are maintained and emotions are preserved.

The diagnosis of dementia is not difficult for those who deal with older people or mental health. The goal of management includes: confirmation of the diagnosis, exclusion of treatable causes by adequate clinical tests and lab investigations, management of medical co-morbidity to reduce their impact on cognitive function, treatment and control of behavioural symptoms, creation of protective environment, appropriate pharmacological intervention, avoidance of unnecessary drugs, use of behavioural interventions and caring of care givers.

Lately, a number of drugs have flooded the market labelled as 'anti-dementing drugs' including ayurvedic preparations. Many of these drugs are useless for treating any kind of dementia. Clinicians and carers will do well to resist the temptation of these drugs indiscriminately as they only increase the cost of treatment for the patient who is also exposed to the side-effects of such drugs, with drug companies being the only beneficiaries.

Barriers to Mental Health Services

Positive mental outlook is essential to healthy ageing. Coping resources and coping strategies to face emotional stresses of late life are largely influenced by value system and cultural traditions. Acknowledgement of mental health problems and willingness to accept mental health interventions and services are also influenced by cultural factors. The existence of mental health problems is often denied because of a few misconceptions: (a) these problems are shameful; (b) a repayment for the bad deeds done in an early life; (c) healing of illnesses is in God's hands; (d) the suffering should be endured; and (e) receiving help indicates loss of control and dignity.

As a result, elderly patients may seek medical care for non-specific somatic complaints such as headache, insomnia, dizziness or other vague physical symptoms instead of seeking psychiatric care. Seeking help from traditional healers is also extremely common for such symptomatology prior to approaching the modern health care system. Thus, the mental health need of older people is greatly underestimated despite very high prevalence of psychiatric illnesses.

Active Ageing: An Achievable Construct

The World Health Organization (WHO) defined active ageing as the process of optimizing opportunities for health, participation and security of older people in order to enhance quality of life as people age.[19] The concept of "active ageing" considers that if ageing is to be a positive experience and longer life is to be accompanied by continuous opportunity for enjoyment and productivity, then ageing must be seen not as a state of "disease and disability" but as a state of "health and fitness". This concept has now been accepted by national organizations, as well as academicians, who support the idea of continued involvement of older people in socially productive and meaningful work. The phrase "active ageing" implies continuous involvement of older people in social, economic, spiritual, cultural and civic activities, and not just the ability of physical movement and survival. Thus, even older people with disease and disability can remain active and contribute to their families, communities and countries.

The determinants of active ageing are: gender and culture, health and social service system, economic factors: income, work and social protection, physical environment, individual's biology, genetics and adaptability, physical activity, healthy eating, abstaining from tobacco and alcohol use and social environment which includes: social support, education, literacy, protection from violence and abuse.

For achievement and enjoyment of active ageing several initiatives are required at individual, societal and governmental levels. These include: (a) reduction in the prevalence of risk factors of serious diseases; (b) adoption of all those factors that protect health and well-being throughout the life-course; (c) development of a health system which emphasizes health promotion, disease prevention and provision of dignified long-term care at an affordable cost; (d) reduction in the burden of illness and disability; (e) improvement in health and enhancement of independence in difficult times by provision of protection to older people; and (f) active participation of older people in all aspects of society.

References

Miller, P.D., S.L. Bonnick, C.J. Rosen, R.D. Altman, L.V. Avioli and J. Dequeker. 2000. "Osteoporosis Prevention, Diagnosis and Therapy". *NIH Consensus Statements*, 17 (1): pp. 1–45.

Shankarn, B. 2000. "Clinical Studies: Incidence of Fracture Neck of Femur and Intertrocahnteric Fractures in Three Delhi Hospitals". *Osteoporosis*, pp. 9–18.

Vita, A.J., R.B. Terry, H.B. Hubert and J.F. Fries. 1998. "Aging, Health Risks, and Cumulative Disability". *The New England Journal of Medicine*, 338: pp. 1035–41.

WHO Technical Report Series 843. 1994. "Assessment of Osteoporotic Fracture Risk and its Role in Screening for Postmenopausal Osteoporosis". Geneva.

3 Cardiovascular Health

Arvind Mathur

Cardiovascular diseases are the primary cause of death in older adults, and among those without clinical disease, high levels of sub-clinical disease are associated with poor survival.[1] Vascular disease is so strongly age-related that it has been proposed as a biomarker of ageing.[2] Studies on "healthy ageing" or "successful ageing" show that those who survive with intact health or function have low levels of modifiable risk factors for common chronic diseases, particularly risk factors for cardiovascular disease.[3–6] Risk factor modification can prevent cardiovascular events and mortality in older adults. *Successful ageing* means remaining free of major, life-threatening chronic disease, i.e., no prior diagnosis of cancer, an absence of cardiovascular disease (CVD) (angina, myocardial infarction, cardiac revascularization procedure, congestive heart failure, stroke, transient ischemic attack, or claudication), no chronic obstructive pulmonary disease (chronic bronchitis, emphysema, or asthma), no reported difficulty with any activities of daily living (ADL), and a modified Mini-Mental State Examination score in the 80th percentile or higher, and having normal physical and cognitive functioning.[7]

Although epidemiological studies have discovered that lipid levels, diabetes, sedentary lifestyle, and genetic factors are risk factors for coronary disease, hypertension, congestive heart failure, and stroke, the quintessential cardiovascular diseases within our society, advancing age unequivocally confers the major risk. The prevalence of these diseases increases steeply with advancing age. Recent studies of sub-clinical cardiovascular disease suggest that some measures to the extent of vascular disease are associated with adverse health effects even in those with no symptoms of vascular disease or history of myocardial infarction, stroke, or other vascular events.[8–9] For example, those with sub-clinical peripheral arterial disease have mobility impairment even without claudication, those with white matter changes on brain magnetic resonance imaging but no history of stroke have demonstrably lower levels of physical performance, and those with sub-clinical disease appear to be more frail.[10–12] These data suggest that sub-clinical cardiovascular disease has adverse effects on health and function and, in addition to causing morbidity from heart disease directly, may contribute to disability and cognitive impairment.

There are several possible explanations for the dominant effect of age on the likelihood for occurrence of these cardiovascular diseases. Increasing age contributes to an increased exposure time to these other age-dependent risk factors. A somewhat different view is that cardiovascular structure and function change with time due to "ageing process," and that, over time, this process alters the substrate on which specific pathophysiological disease mechanisms, such as those that have been linked to experimental atherosclerosis, become superimposed. According to this view, the enhanced risk for older persons to encounter the above diseases is due to age-disease interactions. Age impacts the severity of disease manifestations for a given time at risk. Thus, age-associated changes in cardiovascular structure and function become "partners" with pathophysiological disease mechanisms to determine the threshold, severity, and prognosis of cardiovascular disease occurrence in older persons. However, the true interactions are more complex and involve age, multiple risk factors, and genetics.[13]

To define why age (or an ageing process x exposure time interaction) is a major risk factor for cardiovascular diseases, the specific components of the risk, associated with age, are being looked at. Two complementary approaches have evolved. On the one hand, epidemiologists are searching for novel measures of "sub-clinical disease" (in addition to the more established risk factors that have already been well characterized) in large study cohorts composed of persons both with and without cardiovascular disease. On the other hand, gerontologists are attempting to develop quantitative information on cardiovascular structure and function in apparently healthy individuals to define and target the specific characteristics of ageing that render it such a major risk factor for cardiovascular disease, even in the absence of clinically apparent comorbidity.

Age-associated Changes in Cardiovascular Structures

Arterial Changes

Age-associated changes in the arterial properties of healthy individuals have relevance to the steep age-dependent increase in vascular diseases. With age, arterial wall thickening and dilatation of large elastic arteries, endothelial dysfunction, arterial stiffening, and arterial pulse pressure widening are prominent changes.[14] Combinations of these processes occurring to varying degrees determine the overall vascular ageing profile of a given individual. Additional risk factors, including hypertension, smoking, dyslipidemia, diabetes, diet, and heretofore unidentified genetic factors, interact with vascular ageing to activate an atherosclerotic plaque. These traditional risk factors may themselves accelerate ageing of the vascular wall.

The aortic wall thickening that occurs with ageing consists mainly of intimal media (IM) thickening which is independent of atherosclerosis.[15] There is marked heterogeneity in IM thickness among individuals of a given age. The increased IM thickness is an independent predictor of future cardiovascular events.

Age-associated increase in IM thickening is accompanied by both luminal dilatation and a reduction in compliance or distensibility, with an increase in vessel stiffness. Pulse wave velocity (PWV), a relatively convenient, noninvasive index of vascular stiffening, increases with age both in men and women. The structural alterations in the vascular media include increased collagen, reduced elastin content, elastin fractures, and calcification. The cross-links, due to nonenzymatic glycation, that increase with age and increase markedly in diabetes contribute to age, and disease-related increases in large artery stiffening. However, the stiffness is governed not only by the structural changes within the matrix, as noted above, but also by endothelial regulation of vascular smooth muscle tone and of other aspects of vascular wall structure/function. Thus, there is evidence of a vicious cycle: altered mechanical properties of the vessel wall influence the development of atherosclerosis and the latter, via endothelial cell dysfunction and other mechanisms, influences vascular stiffness.[16]

As the walls of large arteries become stiffer, central systolic arterial pressure increases, diastolic arterial pressure decreases, and the pulse pressure increases for a given pattern of left ventricular ejection. The elevated levels of pulse pressure are associated with progression of IM thickening and that IM thickening, which in turn, is associated with widening of pulse pressure. Numerous studies have concurred that elevated pulse pressure is an independent risk factor for future cardiovascular events.[17–20] Thus, an increased PWV reflects three potential risk factors: increased systolic pressure, widened pulse pressure, and altered vascular wall properties. The elevated pulse wave velocity and reduced total systemic compliance assessed by stroke volume/pulse pressure, over and above blood pressure, are independent predictors of cardiovascular events. This suggests that altered structure/function of the stiff vessel wall, in addition to the associated increase in systolic and pulse pressures, is a risk factor for future vascular events.[21]

In addition to stroke volume, arterial pressure is determined by the interplay of peripheral resistance and central artery stiffness; the former raises both systolic and diastolic pressure to a similar degree, whereas the latter raises systolic but lowers diastolic pressure. Pulse pressure is a useful hemodynamic indicator of conduit artery vascular stiffness. Framingham investigators and others have reported an age-dependent rise in average systolic blood pressure across all adult age groups. In contrast, average diastolic pressure was found to rise until 50 years of age, level off from ages 50 to 60, and decline thereafter. The age-dependent changes in systolic, diastolic, and pulse pressure are consistent with the notion that in younger people, blood pressure is determined largely by peripheral vascular resistance, whereas in older individuals, it is determined to a greater extent by central conduit vessel stiffness.[18–20]

Owing to the decline in diastolic pressure in older men and women in whom systolic pressure is increasing, isolated systolic hypertension emerges as the most common form of hypertension in individuals over the age of 50.[22] Isolated systolic hypertension, even when mild in severity (stage 1), is associated with an appreciable increase in cardiovascular disease risk.[18] Based on long-term follow up of middle-aged and older subjects, however, Framingham researchers have found pulse pressure to be a better predictor of coronary disease risk than the systolic or diastolic pressure.[19] When considered jointly with the systolic blood pressure in older subjects, diastolic blood pressure is inversely related to coronary risk. Consideration of the systolic and diastolic pressures jointly may be preferable to consideration of either value alone.[18,19,22]

Vascular ageing and vascular disease are partners; each contributes specific components to what is presently referred to as "vascular disease." Thus, what clinical medicine and epidemiology now refer to as vascular disease should be regarded as the "vascular ageing-vascular disease interaction."[13] Ageing blood vessels provide the milieu in which vascular diseases can flourish. If vascular ageing is a risk factor for disease, then age-associated vascular changes represent a potential target for treatment and prevention.

Age-associated Changes in Cardiac Structure and Function in Persons Without a Heart Disease Diagnosis

There is a continuum of expression of cardiac structural and functional alterations that occurs with age in healthy humans, and these age-associated cardiac changes seem to have relevance to the steep increases in LVH, chronic heart failure, and AF seen with increasing age.[23]

Cardiac Structure

The left ventricular (LV) wall thickness increases progressively with age in both sexes. Cardiac myocyte enlargement and decrease in the estimated myocyte number was observed at autopsy in older hospitalized patients without apparent cardiovascular disease. An increase in the amount (focal increases) and a change in the physical properties of collagen (purportedly due to nonenzymatic cross-linking) also occur within the myocardium with ageing.

Left Ventricular Diastolic Function

The LV early diastolic filling rate progressively slows after the age of 20 years, so that by 80 years the rate is reduced, on average, up to 50 per cent.[24] Structural (fibrous) changes within the LV myocardium or residual myofilament Ca^{2+} activation from the preceding systole are putative mechanisms for a reduced early diastolic LV filling rate. Despite the slowing of left ventricular filling early in diastole, more filling occurs in late diastole, due, in part, to a more vigorous atrial contraction, which produces an exaggerated A wave. The augmented atrial contraction is accompanied by atrial hypertrophy and enlargement and auscultation is manifested as a fourth heart sound (atrial gallop). Multiple regression analyses indicate that age is the major determinant of the E:A ratio; hence, the age-associated decrease in the Doppler transmittal E:A ratio is identical in healthy Baltimore Longitudinal Study on Aging (BLSA) participants and in Framingham Study participants.[25–26]

Despite the age-associated changes in the diastolic filling pattern in older healthy persons, their left ventricular end-diastolic volume index (end-diastolic volume normalized for body surface area [EDVI]) in the supine position is not compromised and does not substantially differ from their younger counterparts. The altered responses of cardiac volumes to postural manoeuvers are associated with ageing.[27]

Left Ventricular Systolic Function

The LV ejection fraction (EF), the most commonly used clinical measure of LV systolic performance, is preserved during ageing. However, there is an age-associated failure to augment EF with exercise due to a remarkable age-associated deficit in the ability to reduce end-systolic volume index (ESVI); the acute ESV reserve, at age 85, is only about one-fifth of that at age 20, and there is a similar age-associated loss of EF reserve.

The net result of the age-associated changes in EDV and ESV regulation during exercise is that the stroke volume index (SVI) is preserved in these older persons over a wide range of performance demands because of a greater use of the Frank Starling mechanism.

Heart Rate and Cardiac Output

In the supine position at rest, the heart rate (HR) in healthy men does not change with age. With assumption of the seated position from the supine position, HR increases slightly, but significantly less in older than in younger men.[27] The maximum heart rate during exhaustive, dynamic exercise decreases with age, and the magnitude of this age-associated reduction in peak HR is about 30 per cent between 20 and 85 years of age. The reduction in HR response to exercise is the reason why the maximum acute cardiac output reserve in healthy volunteers decreases, on average, by about 30 per cent between ages 20 and 85 years. Healthy individuals at the older end of the age range can augment their cardiac index 2.5–fold over seated rest, whereas those at the younger end of the age spectrum can increase their cardiac index 3.5–fold.

Mechanisms that underlying deficient cardiovascular regulation with ageing in otherwise healthy humans deficits in sympathetic modulation of heart rate and LV contractility.

All of the factors that have been identified as playing a role in deficient cardiovascular regulation with ageing, including HR (and thus filling time), afterload (both cardiac and vascular), myocardial contractility, and redistribution of blood flow, exhibit a deficient sympathetic modulatory component.

Depending on the duration of the stress, enhanced or deficient neurotransmitter release might be a basis for apparent impairment of sympathetic cardiovascular regulation that occurs with ageing.

The age-associated increase in neurotransmitter spillover into the circulation during acute stress implies a greater cellular receptor occupancy by these substances, which leads to desensitization of post-receptor signaling.

Potential age-associated changes in the tissue levels or responses [to growth factors, catecholamines, angiotensin II, endothelin, tumor growth factor ß (TGFß), or fibroblast growth factor (FGF)] that influence myocardial or vascular cells or their extracellular matrices may also have a role.[28]

Left ventricular afterload and vascular-ventricular load matching cardiac afterload has two components, one of which is generated by the heart itself and the other of which is generated by the vasculature. The cardiac component of afterload during exercise can be expected to increase slightly with age because the heart size increases in older persons throughout the cardiac cycle during exercise.[29] The vascular load on the heart has four components: conduit artery compliance characteristics, reflected pulse waves, inertance, and resistance. There is considerable evidence to indicate that each becomes altered during ageing and that at rest, the vascular load on the LV increases with age. Increased vascular loading on the heart is a likely cause of the increase in LV wall thickness associated with ageing.

Optimal and efficient ejection of blood from the heart occurs when ventricular and vascular loads are matched. It has been suggested that the precise cardiac and vascular load matching that is characteristic in younger persons is preserved at older ages, at least at rest, because the increased vascular stiffness in older persons at rest is matched by increased resting ventricular stiffness.[30]

Heart Rhythm

Beat-to-beat fluctuation of HR, commonly known as HR variability, declines steadily with age. Reduced HR variability is an indicator of cardiac autonomic regulation commonly found in older people and has been linked to increased risk for morbid and fatal outcomes.[31]

An increase in the prevalence and complexity of both supraventricular and ventricular arrhythmias, e.g., isolated atrial premature beats (APBs), short bursts of paroxysmal supraventricular tachycardia (PSVT), AF, and ventricular ectopy (VE), whether detected by resting ECG, ambulatory monitoring, or exercise testing, occurs in otherwise healthy older patients but not in younger persons. Neither the prevalence nor the complexity of them is a determinant of future coronary events.

Newman et al. (2003) examined a composite measure of several noninvasive measures of the extent of CVD and then individual measures, including carotid ultrasonogram, ankle-arm index (AAI), and electrocardiogram findings. The composite measure of any sub-clinical disease was defined as presence of any of the following: common or internal carotid wall thickness above the 80th percentile of the distribution for all CHS participants at baseline, maximum per cent stenosis of the internal carotid artery greater than 25 per cent, AAI of 0.9 or less, any major ECG abnormality, or Rose questionnaire findings that were positive for angina or claudication.

Men and women who reach old age in good health without disability or cognitive impairment vary widely in the likelihood of continuing to age successfully. The initial age at study entry was the strongest predictor of continued success, but even within age strata the number of expected years of success was strongly related to other factors, including the extent of sub-clinical vascular disease and health habits. Participants without sub-clinical vascular disease continued to successfully age approximately 5 to 6 years longer than those with sub-clinical disease (women, 6.5 vs men, 5.6 years).[32]

The independent associations of diabetes mellitus, smoking, and physical activity with fewer years of success is important because these risk factors are modifiable. Furthermore, it suggests that their adverse effects on maintaining health and function may be mediated by pathways other than vascular disease. A study in the Honolulu Heart Programme cohort showed that smoking, diabetes mellitus, and hypertension are common factors underlying a composite outcome of successful ageing.[4] Smoking and physical activity were shown to dramatically affect active life expectancy in the MacArthur studies of successful ageing as well.[33] C-reactive protein level and increased physical activity were also associated with successful ageing. Higher CRP levels have previously been documented to predict mortality, CVD, and CVD events in older adults. Inflammation as measured by interleukin 6 has been shown to predict disability, while associations with CRP are less consistent. Factors that predict higher levels of disability include smoking and obesity, but the pathophysiologic basis of these associations is not well defined. Additional work is needed to examine these factors, as well as other factors such as insulin-like growth factor, sex steroid hormones, and homocysteine levels that are hypothesized to affect the ageing process.[34–38]

There are increasing opportunities to identify genetic factors that might affect the age at onset of vascular disease. There is also a growing recognition that there may be protective genetic factors that result in delayed onset of vascular disease, even in the presence of modifiable risk factors such as smoking and cholesterol.[39] Family history also continues to predict vascular disease in late life, and its role is being examined in longevity and successful ageing.

Finally, the potential for the extent of vascular disease to exert its effect on functioning in old age may well be due to its association with a higher rate of disabling cardiovascular events. These analyses suggest that the effects of CVD on functioning are sub-clinical in that the associations persisted even when disease was excluded from the outcome and intervening events were accounted for.

Improving the quality of late life and maintaining intact health and function are important public health goals. Prevention of CVD should be a major priority for the achievement of successful ageing. If the burden of vascular disease is shifted to later in life, the age-related trajectory of decline would be attenuated by several years. Current treatments for cardiovascular risk factors, including smoking cessation, lipid lowering, blood pressure treatment, and avoidance of obesity through diet and exercise, are underutilized. Recent recommendations for risk factor modification suggest that markers of the extent of sub-clinical vascular disease may be useful to target intervention in older adults, especially those without elevations in cardiovascular risk factors.[40]

Lifestyle intervention or pharmacotherapy to retard the rate of progression of sub-clinical disease might be considered before the clinical disease becomes manifest. Lifestyle changes are an effective approach to CV prevention. Patient education and counselling on nonpharmacologic preventive strategies like moderate exercise, proper diet, weight reduction and smoking cessation is useful.

With respect to lifestyle, the risk factor of lack of vigorous exercise increases dramatically with age in otherwise healthy persons. It is noteworthy that pulse pressure, PWV, and carotid augmentation index are lower and baroreceptor reflex function is improved in older persons who are physically conditioned compared with sedentary persons.[41] Exercise conditioning also improves endothelial function in older persons.

Preventive pharmacotherapies are efficacious and cost effective in the older population. Antiplatelet therapy, ACE inhibitors, beta-blocker therapy, and cholesterol lowering drugs (statins) have shown to reduce CV risk. The cumulative impact of these four cardioprotective medication classes in post-MI patients is about 70 per cent.[42]

Despite the demonstrated benefits of polypharmacy in the prevention of CV events, possible adverse effects and drug interactions must be considered whenever prescribing multiple agents in the older persons. Older patients often are receiving a number of drugs for the treatment of various conditions common with ageing. With concomitant medication use comes the increased potential for drug interactions and cumulative adverse effects. In elderly it is essential to evaluate complete medication profile, to eliminate any unneeded drugs and to use lowest effective dose of all agents to maintain effectiveness and promote safety and tolerability.

Notes

1. L.H. Kuller, L. Shemanski, B.M. Psaty et al. "Subclinical disease as an independent risk factor for cardiovascular disease". *Circulation.* 1995; 92: 720–726.
2. S.M. Grundy. "Age as a risk factor: You are as old as your arteries". *American Journal of Cardiology.* 1999; 83: 1455–1457.
3. J.W. Rowe and R.L. Kahn. "Human aging: Usual and successful". *Science.* 1987; 237: 143–149.
4. D.W. Reed, D.J. Foley, L.R. White, H. Heimovitz, C.M. Burchfiel and K. Masaki. "Predictors of healthy aging in men with high life expectancies". *American Journal of Public Health.* 1998; 88: 1463–1468.
5. T.E. Seeman, P.A. Charpentier, L.F. Berkman et al. "Predicting changes in physical performance in a high-functioning elderly cohort: MacArthur studies of successful aging". *The Journal of Gerontology.* 1994; 49: M97–M108.
6. G.L. Burke, A.M. Arnold, D.E. Bild et al. CHS Collaborative Research Group. "Factors associated with healthy aging: The Cardiovascular Health Study". *Journal of American Geriatrics Society.* 2001; 49: 254–262.
7. M.B. Mittelmark, B.M. Psaty, P.M. Rautaharju et al. "Prevalence of cardiovascular diseases among older adults: The Cardiovascular Health Study". *American Journal of Epidemiol.* 1993; 137: 311–317.
8. D.H. O'Leary, J.F. Polak, R.A. Kronmal, T.A. Manolio, G.L. Burke and S.K. Wolfson. Cardiovascular Health Study Collaborative Research Group. "Carotid-artery intima and media thickness as a risk factor for myocardial

infarction and stroke in older adults". *The New England Journal of Medicine (NEJM)*. 1999; 340: 14–22.

9. L.H. Kuller, P. Velentgas, J. Barzilay, N. Beauchamp, D.H. O'Leary and P.J. Savage. "Diabetes mellitus: Subclinical cardiovascular disease and risk of incident cardiovascular disease and all-cause mortality". *Arterioscler Thromb Vasc Biol.* 2000; 20: 823–829.
10. M.M. McDermott, S.M. Ohlmiller, L. Kiang et al. "Gait alterations associated with walking impairment in people with peripheral arterial disease with and without intermittent claudication". *Journal of American Geriatrics Society.* 2001; 49: 747–754.
11. W.T. Longstreth, T.A. Manolio, A. Arnold et al. Cardiovascular Health Study Collaborative Research Group. "Clinical correlates of white matter findings on cranial magnetic resonance imaging of 3301 elderly people". *Stroke.* 1996; 27: 1274–1282.
12. A.B. Newman, J.S. Gottdiener, M.A. McBurnie et al. Cardiovascular Health Study Research Group. "Associations of subclinical cardiovascular disease with frailty". *J Gerontol A Biol Sci Med Sci.* 2001; 56: M158–M166.
13. E.G. Lakatta and D. Levy. "Arterial and cardiac aging: Major shareholders in cardiovascular disease enterprises. Part I: Aging arteries: A "set up" for vascular disease". *Circulation.* 2003; 107: 139–146.
14. E.G. Lakatta. "Cardiovascular regulatory mechanisms in advanced age". *Physiological Reviews.* 1993; 73: 413–465.
15. R. Virmani, A.P. Avolio, W.J. Mergner et al. "Effect of aging on aortic morphology in populations with high and low prevalence of hypertension and atherosclerosis: Comparison between occidental and Chinese communities". *American Journal of Pathology.* 1991; 139: 1119–1129. [Abstract]
16. J. Blacher, R. Asmar, S. Djane et al. "Aortic pulse wave velocity as a marker of cardiovascular risk in hypertensive patients". *Hypertension.* 1999; 33: 1111–1117.
17. A.M. Dart and B.A. Kingwell. "Pulse pressure: A review of mechanisms and clinical relevance". *Journal of American College of Cardiology.* 2001; 37: 975–984.
18. S.S. Franklin, M.G. Larson, S.A. Khan et al. "Does the relation of blood pressure to coronary heart disease risk change with aging? The Framingham Heart Study". *Circulation.* 2001; 103: 1245–1249.
19. S.S. Franklin, S.A. Khan, N.D. Wong et al. "Is pulse pressure useful in predicting risk for coronary heart disease? The Framingham Heart Study". *Circulation.* 1999; 100: 354–360.
20. S.S. Franklin, William Gustin IV and N.D. Wong et al. "Hemodynamic patterns of age-related changes in blood pressure. The Framingham Heart Study". *Circulation.* 1997; 96: 308–315.

21. P. Boutouyrie, A.I. Tropeano, R. Asmar et al. "Aortic stiffness is an independent predictor of primary coronary events in hypertensive patients: A longitudinal study". *Hypertension.* 2002; 39: 10–15.
22. A. Sagie, M.G. Larson and D. Levy. "The natural history of borderline isolated systolic hypertension". *NEJM.* 1993; 329: 1912–1917.
23. E.G. Lakatta and D. Levy. "Arterial and cardiac aging: Major shareholders in cardiovascular disease enterprises. Part II: The aging heart in health: Links to heart disease". *Circulation*. 2003; 107: 346–354.
24. S. Schulman, E.G. Lakatta, J.L. Fleg et al. "Age-related decline in left ventricular filling at rest and exercise". *American Journal of Physiology.* 1992; 263: H1932–H1938.
25. E.J. Benjamin, D. Levy, K.M. Anderson et al. "Determinants of Doppler indexes of left ventricular diastolic function in normal subjects (the Framingham Heart Study)". *American Journal Cardiology.* 1992; 70: 508–515.
26. C.J. Swinne, E.P. Shapiro, S.D. Lima et al. "Age-associated changes in left ventricular diastolic performance during isometric exercise in normal subjects". *American Journal Cardiology.* 1992; 69: 823–826.
27. R.J. Rodeheffer, G. Gerstenblith, E. Beard et al. "Postural changes in cardiac volumes in men in relation to adult age". *Experimental Gerontology on Science Direct.* 1986; 21: 367–378.
28. E.G. Lakatta. "Cardiovascular regulatory mechanisms in advanced age". *Physiological Reviews.* 1993; 73: 413–465.
29. J.L. Fleg, F.C. O'Connor, G. Gerstenblith et al. "Impact of age on the cardiovascular response to dynamic upright exercise in healthy men and women". *Journal of Applied Physiology.* 1995; 78: 890–900.
30. C.H. Chen, M. Nakayama, M. Talbot et al. "Verapamil acutely reduces ventricular-vascular stiffening and improves aerobic exercise performance in elderly individuals". *Journal of American Colloege of Cardiology.* 1999; 33: 1602–1609.
31. H. Tsuji, M.G. Larson, F.J. Venditti et al. "Impact of reduced heart rate variability on risk for cardiac events". *Circulation.* 1996; 94: 2850–2855.
32. A.B. Newman, A.M. Arnold, B.L. Naydeck et al. "Successful Aging: Effect of Subclinical Cardiovascular Disease". *Archives of International Medicine.* 2003; 163: 2315–2322.
33. L. Ferrucci, G. Izmirlian, S. Leveille et al. "Smoking, physical activity, and active life expectancy". *American Journal of Epidemiology.* 1999; 149: 645–653.
34. T.B. Harris, L. Ferrucci, R.P. Tracy et al. "Associations of elevated interleukin-6 and C-reactive protein levels with mortality in the elderly". *The American Journal of Medicine.* 1999; 106: 506–512.

35. P.M. Ridker, R.J. Glynn and C. Hennekens. "C-reactive protein adds to the predictive value of total and HDL cholesterol in determining risk of first myocardial infarction". *Circulation.* 1998; 97: 2007–2011.

36. L. Ferrucci, T.B. Harris, J.M. Guralnik et al. "Serum IL-6 level and the development of disability in older persons". *Journal of American Geriatrics Society.* 1999; 47: 639–646.

37. J. Walston, M.A. McBurnie, A. Newman et al. Cardiovascular Health Study. "Frailty and activation of the inflammation and coagulation systems with and without clinical comorbidities: Results from the Cardiovascular Health Study". *Archives of International Medicine.* 2002; 162: 2333–2341.

38. M. Pahor and S. Kritchevsky. "Research hypotheses on muscle wasting, aging, loss of function and disability". *Journal of Nutrition Health and Aging.* 1998; 2: 97–100.

39. O. Stein, J. Thiery and Y. Stein. "Is there a genetic basis for resistance to atherosclerosis?" *Atherosclerosis.* 2002; 160: 1–10.

40. P. Greenland, S.C. Smith and S.M. Grundy. "Improving coronary heart disease risk assessment in asymptomatic people: Role of traditional risk factors and noninvasive cardiovascular tests". *Circulation.* 2001; 104: 1863–1867.

41. P.V. Vaitkevicius, J.L. Fleg, J.H. Engel et al. "Effects of Age and Aerobic capacity on arterial stiffness in healthy adults". *Circulation.* 1993; 88: 1456–1462.

42. T.A. Pearson, S.N. Blair, S.R. Daniels et al. "AHA Guidelines for Primary Prevention of Cardiovascular Disease and Stroke: 2002 Update". *Circulation.* 2002; 106: 338–391.

4 Diabetics

D. Dalus

Epidemiology

It is projected that by 2010 the number of diabetic individuals in the world will reach 221 million, compared with 151 million in 2000. This increase in prevalence can be attributed to several important risk factors such as advancing age of the population, greater number of people from ethnic minority backgrounds adopting a "transitional" lifestyle, greater levels of overweight and obesity, and more sedentary lifestyles.

Diabetes care systems for older people require an integrated approach between general practitioners, hospital specialists, and other members of the health care team. This should be multidimensional, with an emphasis on prevention of diabetes and its complications, early intervention for vascular disease, and assessment of disability due to limb problems, eye disease and stroke.

Type 2 diabetes mellitus is a common disabling chronic medical disorder that has a tremendous health, social and economic burden. One therapeutic approach, to the management of type 2 diabetes in ageing subjects, is to concentrate on strategies designed to limit and ameliorate both defective insulin secretion and insulin resistance. The term *metabolic syndrome* now embraces the view that type 2 diabetes represents a cluster of cardiovascular risk factors which in turn represent a significant vascular threat. In older subjects, the added effects of ageing and renal impairment increase the impact of this syndrome. Some of the features may be present up to 10 years before the onset of overt hyperglycemia, thus increasing the cardiovascular risk before the onset of diabetes.

Management of diabetes in older people can be relatively straightforward especially when patients have no other comorbidities and when vascular complications are absent. In many cases, however, special issues arise which increase the complexity of management and lead to difficult clinical decision making. Diabetes in older subjects is characterized by a series of factors that highlight deficiencies in care and tend to increase the complexity of management.

Characteristics of Older Subjects with Diabetes

- Common comorbidities of diabetes.
- Age-related impairment of functional ability.
- Increased vulnerability to hypoglycemia.
- Age-specific complications.
- Increased mortality from acute metabolic decompenzation.
- Poor medial follow-up by primary-care physicians, diabetic specialists, and geriatricians.
- Need to involve spouses and informal carers in management.

Modes of Presentation

Presentation of diabetes in older people is often varied and may be insidious, which ultimately delays diagnosis. Many cases are detected by noting hyperglycemia during hospital admissions for other co morbidities or acute illnesses. Even when hyperglycemia has been recognized in hospital about half the subjects receive no further evaluation for diabetes or treatment. Some patients do not have the classic features of either diabetic ketoacidosis or hyperosmolar nonketotic coma but present with a "mixed" disturbance of hyperglycemia (blood glucose levels 15–25 mM; arterial blood pH of 7.2 or 7.3, not particularly acidotic), and without marked dehydration or change in level of consciousness.

Recognition of the symptom profile of hyperglycemia in older subjects can be helpful in making an early diagnosis but the atypical presentation and diverse effects of this metabolic disorder make it difficult.

Varying Presentation of Diabetes in Older People

Asymptomatic (coincidental finding) Classical osmotic symptoms metabolic disturbances	Diabetic ketoacidosis Hyperosmolar non-ketotic coma "Mixed" metabolic disturbance
Spectrum of vague symptoms	Depressed mood Apathy Mental confusion
Development of "geriatric" syndromes	Falls or poor mobility muscle weakness, vision, cognitive impairment Urinary incontinence Unexplained weight loss, memory disorder or cognitive impairment
Slow recovery from specific illnesses or increased vulnerability	Impaired recovery from stroke repeated infections, Poor wound healing

Diabetic Retinopathy and Visual Loss

The majority of older patients with diabetes will have diabetic retinopathy of some description although about one in twenty show no evidence of retinal damage even after 15 years. Factors that were significantly associated with visual loss in diabetic subjects included advanced age, female sex, history of foot ulceration, duration of diabetes, and treatment with insulin.

The underlying problem in diabetic retinopathy is capillary occlusion; this may cause retinal hypoxia and increased vascular permeability, with new vessel formation secondary to vascular endothelial growth factor production. However, other capillaries become dilated, which causes micro aneurysms (if focal or leakage from the capillaries is generalized). It is this capillary leakage that causes exudative and edematous maculopathies, which are the main forms of sight-threatening retinopathy in the older patients with type 2 diabetes.

The Diabetes Control and Complications Trial (DCCT) in type I diabetes and the United Kingdom Prospective Diabetes Study (UKPDS) in type 2 diabetes has demonstrated convincingly that tight control of hyperglycemia leads to a reduction in retinopathy. Unfortunately, there are no specific intervention studies in elderly type 2 diabetes subjects. The UKPDS demonstrated a 25 per cent rise reduction in retinopathy when tight control was present (HbA1C<7.0%). Duration of disease is also associated with increased risk of retinopathy. Achieving a target systolic blood pressure of <140 mmHg in the UKPDS, a 37 per cent reduced rate of progression of retinopathy was demonstrated providing support for the additional benefits of blood pressure control. Diabetes retinopathy is already present at diagnosis in 23.8 per cent of subject of all ages in the UKPDS.

Without laser intervention in proliferative diabetic retinopathy, the risk of severe visual loss is 50–70 per cent at 2 and 5 years. Laser photocoagulation can preserve vision in edematous (reduces risk of visual deterioration by 50 per cent and exudative maculopathies if visual acuity is 6/9 or better, and it has been calculated that screening and treating diabetic retinopathy would prevent 56 per cent of blind registrations due to this condition. Cataract is the most common cause of deteriorating vision in the elderly population and has been shown to be more common in diabetes subjects, even at the time of diagnosis, and its presence suggests increased future mortality.

Age-related macular degeneration is common in diabetic patients and its prevalence will increase with age. It is an important cause of central vision loss. Risk factors include atherosclerosis, diastolic blood pressure>95 mmHg, antihypertensive medication, and elevated serum cholesterol.

Screening for retinopathy in the elderly is particularly important as deteriorating vision may not be regarded as a significant event by the subject who expects "age-related" changes. Retinopathy may be the presenting feature of diabetes in older people, and a screening tool using digital fundus photography is being developed. If photography is not available, subjects need measurements of visual acuity and dilated fundoscopy by experienced observers each year. In the absence of poor metabolic control and/or hypertension, some ophthalmologists may accept an interval of 2–3 years. This is probably worth doing anyway, opportunistically, as even photography misses 11 per cent of retinopathy. Although exudative maculopathy is easy to spot in the dilated eye (exudates around or within I disc's diameter of the macula), macular edema is practically impossible to distinguish from a normal eye by ophthalmoscopy, hence the importance of measuring the corrected visual younger counterparts. But the threshold for referral may vary.

Diabetic Foot Syndrome

Amputation of a limb remains an important and expensive health problem in the diabetic population, with the elderly being particularly affected. A recent study from the Netherlands identified increasing age and a higher level of amputation as important factors leading to increases in the duration of hospitalization with its associated cost, and to increases in the number of deaths.

The 3-year survival following lower extremity amputation is about 50 per cent, and in about 70 per cent of cases, amputation is precipitated by foot ulceration. The principal antecedents include peripheral vascular disease, sensorimotor and autonomic neuropathy, limited joint mobility (which impairs the ability of older people to inspect their feet), and high foot pressures. The majority of the elderly diabetic population is at increased risk of developing foot ulcers. Factors that have been identified as increasing the likelihood of foot ulceration are shown. Peripheral sensorimotor neuropathy is the primary cause or contributory factor in the vast majority of cases. This may cause common symptoms of numbness, lancinating and burning pain, pins and needles, and hyperesthesia (which is typically worse at night), and evidence of high foot pressures leading to gait disturbances, falls and other foot injuries. The presence of visual loss increases the consequences of this situation. A trivial foot injury in a patient with severe neuropathy can eventually lead to the development of a Charcot's joint; the majority of cases have had diabetes for at least 10 years and most are elderly.

Treatment of painful neuropathy in older patients is often difficult but may improve with better metabolic control, in pain which is of recent onset. Pain associated with a loss of sensation and lasting longer than six months requires specific therapy. Patients with localized pain may respond to a topical cream called capsaicin (0.075%). which works by depleting the neurotransmitter, substance P). Alternative treatment includes transcutaneous nerve stimulation or acupuncture. Drug therapies include tricyclic antidepressants and antiepileptics such as carbamazepine although these are given off-license by some physicians. Lower doses are recommended initially for older patients but in the presence of cardiac disease, e.g., arrhythmias, TCADs are not advised, and with carbamazepine, a history of cardiac, renal, or hepatic disease may not allow its use. Gabapentin has recently been licensed for the treatment of painful neuropathy. A recent review of five randomized clinical trials examining the effects of gabapentin in managing the pain of diabetic neuropathy found that the drug relieved the symptoms of allodynia, burning pain, shooting pain, and hyperesthesia, at a dosage of 1800–3600 mg/day with reasonably good tolerance.

Risk Factors for Foot Ulceration in the Elderly

- Peripheral sensorimotor neuropathy
- Automatic: neuropathy
- Peripheral vascular disease
- Limited joint mobility
- Foot pressure abnormalities including deformity
- Previous foot problems
- Visual loss

History of Alcohol Abuse

Both the micro and macro circulations are disturbed in diabetic limbs. Some of these abnormalities may be reversible, or ameliorated by improved glycemic control. Chronic change in peripheral blood vessels is usually manifested by atherosclerosis with the pattern of PVD tending to involve vessels below the knee more often in diabetic than in nondiabetic individuals. Risk factors for PVD include smoking, hypertension, and dyslipidemia, with prevalence increasing with both advancing age and duration of diabetes. Symptoms include intermittent claudication and/or rest pain, with lower limb ulceration or gangrene being important clinical outcomes. Radiological investigation may show medial arterial calcification and this may be associated with both diabetic peripheral somatosensory and autonomic neuropathy. Objective assessment of limb blood flow by Doppler ultrasound can be affected by extensive medial calcification, giving rise to a misleadingly high ankle-pressure index. An appropriate and early referral for vascular assessment is mandatory in elderly patients with PVD who may benefit from arterial reconstruction or angioplasty. This is best organized through joint protocols developed by the diabetes specialist and the vascular surgeon. A reasonable life expectancy is considered important by surgeons since concomitant cardiac and cerebrovascular disease may account for death in 50 per cent of cases within 5 years.

Interventions designed to prevent diabetic foot disease and amputations should be directed to the prevention of peripheral neuropathy and PVD, including the prevention, early detection, and treatment of foot lesions. Several studies using staff and patient education, and a multidisciplinary approach to foot care, have demonstrated a reduction in diabetes-related amputations. In proximal arterial reconstruction the 5-year patency averages 70 per cent, and in those patients with high co morbidity levels, graft patency may exceed life expectancy: for distal reconstruction surgery, 5-year limb salvage rates approach 85 per cent.

For many elderly patients having great difficulty in performing the most routine foot care, often as a result of poor vision and reduced mobility, it becomes very important that strategies are designed which enable both spouses and other carers to have a role in the preventive treatment of foot lesions. Educational material needs to be concise and repeated regularly. Video presentations may also be helpful.

Erectile Dysfunction

Erectile dysfunction (ED) due to diabetes in older adults is age-related, and occurs earlier and more commonly than in the general population. At least three important studies indicate the importance of ED in older people which is often neglected and may be an obvious reason for a diminished quality of life or depressive illness. After the age of 60 years, 95 per cent of diabetic men are affected, while the corresponding figure for non-diabetic counterparts is 50 per cent. The etiology of ED, defined as the inability to attain and maintain an erection satisfactory for sexual intercourse, is a complex problem involving several mechanisms. Vasculopathy, autonomic neuropathy, hormonal dysregulation, endothelial dysfunction, and psychogenic factors have all been implicated. Drug-related causes may be a particular problem in older patients, with thiazide diuretics, cimetidine, blockers and spironolactone especially being implicated. A comprehensive history, full medical examination, blood testing for diabetes control, and lipids, testosterone, and thyroid function tests are necessary. Other more sophisticated tests are available through diabetes ED clinics in most large centres, and may involve testing for prolactin, other gonadotrophins and for nocturnal penile tumescence. For many older patients, extensive testing is often avoided. As treatment is available for some patients, e.g., oral Sildenafil (achieved erections were possible in 67 per cent of elderly men in one study).

Metabolic Coma

Diabetic ketoacidosis (DKA) and hyperglycemic hyperosmolar nonketotic (HONK) comas also occur in older subjects with diabetics. HONK comas are predominant in subjects aged over 50 years. Compared with the young, older subjects with hyperglycemic comas have a higher mortality. Those who have had diabetes diagnosed previously are more likely to have renal impairment, and require a greater amount of insulin as treatment.

It appears that in hyperglycemic comas most subjects with type 2 diabetes have little insulin, just enough to suppress lipolysis and ketogenesis, thus avoiding DKA, and develop a HONK coma instead. The tendency to hyperosmolality in HONK comas may be worsened in elderly people, who may not appreciate thirst well, may have difficulty in drinking enough to compensate for their osmotic diuresis, and may also be on diuretics. It also appears that hyperosmolality not only worsens insulin resistance but may also inhibit lipolysis.

Death may be due to the metabolic disturbance and to acute illnesses such as pneumonia and myocardial infarction. The cause of the hyperglycemia may be infection, infarction, inadequate hypoglycemic treatment, or inappropriate drug treatment.

Treatment of Hyperglycemic Comas

The patient history and examination should focus on previous medication, evidence of heart failure, and the degree of dehydration. Initial investigations are as for younger patients, but it is essential to measure arterial blood gases. Attention to pressure areas is essential and monitoring of renal function paramount in an older patient.

Each major hospital unit will have an agreed fluid and insulin and potassium replacement protocol to use in these cases. Intravenous fluid replacement at a rate of 500 ml/h over the initial 4 hours, reduced to 250 ml/h afterwards, should take place. The patient needs more rapid infusion if he or she is shocked, and here a central line is invaluable for monitoring quick infusions, particularly in the presence of cardiac failure or recent myocardial infarction.

Older subjects with a HONK coma may need very small doses of insulin to reduce plasma glucose levels; however, if the patient is catabolic or has marked insulin resistance, larger doses of insulin may be required. Thrombotic complications may occur, or may well have occurred before hospitalization, in subjects with a HONK coma. A prophylactic regimen should be considered.

Older People and Hypoglycemia

In older patients, susceptibility to hypoglycemia is pronounced, and this is exacerbated by old people having little knowledge about the symptoms and signs of hypoglycemia. Indeed, health professionals may misdiagnose hypoglycemia as a stroke or transient ischemic attack, unexplained confusion, or epileptic fit.

Hypoglycemia with Sulfonylurea

An important clinical problem for older subjects taking glibenclamide and chlorpropamide is prolonged hypoglycemia, especially when many older people have so little knowledge of the symptoms of hypoglycemia. Glibenclamide-induced hypoglycemia may be more pronounced because the drug accumulates within β-cells and its metabolites retain some hypoglycemic activity.

It should be remembered that insulin therapy carries a greater risk of hypoglycemia than do sulfonylurea but the introduction of insulin analogues may decrease this risk. Newer oral agents such as the glitazones and the meglitinides may also lower the risk of hypoglycemia in the elderly. In the elderly, serious hypoglycemia appears to have a worse prognosis with high mortality following hospital admission; some patients who survive may have permanent neurological damage, presumably because of a cerebral circulation. Most sulfonylurea have caused fatal hypoglycemia, although this is often associated with chlorpropamide or glibenclamide. Other factors apart from old age that predispose to fatal hypoglycemia are alcohol consumption, poor food intake, renal impairment, potentiation of hypoglycemia by other drugs, and prescription of sulfonylureas. Many, if not all, of these factors are directly relevant in the elderly patient with type 2 diabetes.

Cognitive Impairment, Dementia and Diabetes

Impaired cognitive function has been demonstrated in elderly subjects with diabetes, but these studies were generally not population based, excluded subjects with dementia, and generally used large battery of tests to show the deficit. Community-based studies in Melton Mowbray, Nottingham, and South Wales have shown worse cognitive function in elderly diabetic subjects, using simple tests.

Impaired glucose tolerance has also been shown to be associated with cognitive dysfunction. It has been suggested that many of the deficits seen in the metabolic syndromes (hyperglycemia, dyslipidemia, and hypertension) may each play a role in memory disturbance in type 2 diabetes, and increased serum insulin may be associated with decreased cognitive function and dementia in women.

Cognitive dysfunction in older diabetic subjects has considerable implications which include increased hospitalization, less ability for self-care, less likelihood of specialist follow-up, and increased risk of institutionalization. Impaired cognitive function should he borne in mind when treating elderly diabetic patients as it has implications for their safe treatment. It may cause difficulty with glycemic control due to erratic diet and medications, and may present as hypoglycemia if the patient forgets that he or she has taken the hypoglycemic medication and repeats the dose.

Depression and Diabetes

Major depressive disorder increases significantly the risk of diabetes, and in another study diabetes was significantly associated with depression, independent of age, gender, or presence of chronic disease. The presence of depression was the single most important indicator of subsequent death in a group of diabetic patients admitted into hospital. Failure to recognize depression can be serious since it is a long term, life threatening, disabling illness that can have a significant impact on quality of life. Depression may be associated with worsening diabetic control and decreased treatment compliance.

There is a relative lack of specific evidence linking neuroendocrine abnormalities with diabetes. At this stage, the probable explanation is that depression is due to the effect of the increased stress and strain of having a chronic medical condition in a susceptible individual. Diabetes and depression share similar symptomatology, for example, fatigue, irritability, and sexual dysfunction, and this may delay or confuse the diagnosis. However, commonly used diagnostic assessment scales are unlikely to be greatly affected by these overlapping symptoms. In routine practice, enquire about well-being, sleep, appetite, and weight loss as part of the assessment of older patients with diabetes. If alerted, take a more comprehensive psychiatric evaluation and use a geriatric depression scale score (>5) as indicative of probable depression. Treatment with serotonin selective reuptake inhibitors (SSRIs) such as fluoxetine may improve symptoms with a consequent improvement in metabolic control.

Issues in Treatment and Care

Making the Diagnosis

An early diagnosis may reduce morbidity (detection and prevention of vascular complications) and cardiovascular mortality, although evidence for this is lacking. The diagnostic criteria are identical in young and old patients but some concern has been expressed about the applicability of a fasting glucose level for diagnosis in many older patients, and mortality may be higher in those patients diagnosed as diabetic with the 2-h glucose value than the new fasting criteria alone. In addition, isolated post load hyperglycemia with normal fasting glucose (7.0 mmol/L) is associated with increased fatal cardiovascular disease and heart disease in elderly women.

Many patients may not be able to give an accurate history of symptoms; classic hyperosmolar symptoms of polyuria and polydipsia may be absent because of a combination of altered thirst sensation and a variable renal threshold for glycosuria. A true fasted sample may be difficult to obtain and may be normal in any case, and an oral glucose tolerance test (OGTT) may be thought of as time-consuming and inconvenient. In some cases, elderly patients have elevated plasma glucose levels, which are secondary to acute illness, diabetogenic therapy, or other stress-inducing disorders. Most cases will be diagnosed without the need for an OGTT but this should be employed where doubt exists. The demonstration of an elevated HbA1C in this situation is a pointer to the likely presence of diabetes. Retesting following an acute illness may sometimes prevent false diagnosis being made.

Initial Management

The principal aims of managing diabetes in older adults are given below. The priority of each may be provisionally established at an early stage but may change with disease duration, development of complications, and need for external help. Self-monitoring by patients or carers should be encouraged as part of an empowerment and educational approach to improving self-care activities.

For those presenting with type 2 diabetes, in a non-acute presentation, four important steps are needed: establish the diagnosis of diabetes; screen for vascular complications and assess cardiovascular risk; assess the ability of the patient for diabetes self-care: and initiate treatment. An important aspect of care relates to producing an initial diabetes care plan. No specific stepwise algorithm has been adopted for treatment and the guidelines of the International Diabetes Federation are equally applicable for older subjects. In this section we shall limit our discussion to the management of diabetes in older people.

Major Aims in Managing Older People with Diabetes

Medical	*Patient-orientated*
Freedom from hyper glycemic symptoms	Maintain general well-being and good quality of life
Prevent undesirable weight loss	Acquire skills and knowledge to make lifestyle changes
Avoid hypoglycemia and other adverse reactions	Encourage diabetes self-care
Screen for and prevent vascular complications	
Detect cognitive impairment and depression at an early stage	
Achieve a normal life expectancy for patients where possible	

Care Plan for the Initial Management of Diabetes

1. Establish realistic glycemic and blood pressure targets.
2. Ensure consensus with patient, spouse or family, general practitioner, informal caretaker, community nurse or hospital specialist
3. Define the frequency and nature of diabetes follow-up.
4. Organize glycernic monitoring by patient or carer.
5. Refer to social or community services as necessary.

Initial Treatment

Dietary measures and lifestyle advice is given as for middle-aged subjects, irrespective of the presentation. This represents a low risk but potentially high-benefit strategy. In some cases, a specified exercise programme is instituted. These may be sufficient for those subjects whose initial random glucose levels are less than 15 mmol/I, and in whom symptoms are minimal. If metabolic targets are not reached by 6–8 weeks, oral therapy is usually required. Strict glycemic targeting approaches are possible for many older subjects. However, a reasonable view applicable to patients with single system involvement (free of other major comorbidities) is to aim for control as follows: a fasting glucose range of 5–7 mmol/I (depending on their ability to self-care) and a random level of 6–9 mmol/I. A glycosylated hemoglobin (HbA1c) range of 6.5–7.5 per cent is also recommended but increases the risk of hypoglycemia. For frail subjects (dependent, multisystem disease, care home residency including those with dementia), a fasting glucose of 7–9 mmol/I and a HbA1c range of 7.5–8.5 per cent should be aimed for. In general, both sets of targets should reduce the occurrence of hyperglycemic malaise and the stricter target should have some preventative benefits in terms of vascular complication rate. Attention to lipid and blood pressure targets is essential to complement these approaches.

Glucose Regulation: Use of Oral Agents in Type 2 Diabetes in Old Age

Sulfonylureas

These are often felt to be the oral agent of choice for the elderly diabetic patient, who is failing to comply with diet recommendations, because they are generally well tolerated (apart from their risk of hypoglycemia) without substantial risk of gastrointestinal upset associated with other oral agents. They can achieve a fall of HbA1C of about 1.5 per cent. Glibenclamide appears particularly likely to cause hypoglycemia and its use has been associated with fatalities more than do other sulfonylureas including chlorpropamide. Glibenclamide should be strictly avoided. Gliclazide has a relatively low risk of hypoglycemia and it may be less likely to cause weight gain, the other common problem with sulfonylureas. It is undoubtedly safer than glibenclamide. If hypoglycemia is a major worry, then tolbutamide has the lowest risk, and this may be used in those with renal impairment. If compliance is a problem, then glimepiride is useful since the tablet range means that the dose for all patients is one tablet before breakfast; however, there are no good comparisons between this and gliclazide. Alternatively, a modified release preparation of gliclazide is now available.

Metformin

Metformin is predictable and safe if used correctly, but there are contra-indications to its use: these include renal impairment (creatinine >120 mmol/l), hepatic or cardiac failure, critical limb ischemia, any acute illness, and the use of intravenous radiological contrast media. As a result, often about 40–50 per cent of older subjects may be ineligible for use of metformin. Particular advantages of metformin are that it does not cause hypoglycemia on its own, it does not cause weight gain, and it is inexpensive. Its therapeutic benefits are similar to those with sulfonylureas, and in the UKPDS all cause mortality and any diabetes-related endpoint were significantly lower on intensive treatment with metformin than with insulin or sulfonylurea in obese subjects. It has been shown to be an effective treatment for the elderly, with results similar to those with tolbutarnide. The usual daily dose required is approximately 1.7 g, and it is as effective in the lean as in the overweight, and lowers HbA1C by 1.5 per cent. An extended-release form has the advantage of once-daily dosing.

The FDA in the United States limits the use of metformin to patients aged less than 80 years (unless they have normal renal function), presumably because of their increased risk of lactic acidosis; other side effects include gastrointestinal disturbance, which is minimized by gentle introduction of the agent. Metformin may also cause vitamin B_{12} malabsorption; hence, it is wise to check B_{12} level every 5 years.

An insulin secretagogue should be used in combination with metformin in overweight patients (BMI > 25 kg/m^2) where glycemic targets have not been achieved or maintained.

Acarbose

Since only 1–2 per cent of oral Acarbose is absorbed, it is relatively free of major systemic side effects and its main contraindications are inflammatory bowel disease and sub-acute obstruction. Acarbose can be successfully combined with metformin, sulfonylureas, or insulin. It's not as effective as other oral agents in older subjects.

Thiazolidinediones

These reduce insulin resistance by activating the peroxisome proliferator activated receptor gamma (PPAR-y). They do not cause hypoglycemia and the only problems seem to be weight gain, mild edema, and anaemia (in less than 5% of subjects). Although clinical trials did include subjects with New York Heart Association heart failure grade 2 and no patient developed acute left ventricular failure, they are contraindicated in heart failure (and consequently are not to be used with insulin at the present time). They are safe in mild to moderate renal impairment. They have the potential to cause liver function abnormalities and frequent monitoring of liver function is required especially during the first 12 months of treatment; this is an important disadvantage for many older patients.

They can be used as monotherapy (although not all countries have a monotherapy license), combined with metformin or sulfonylurea, or combined with insulin (where license permits). They can be used as once daily medications and an HbA1C fall of about 0.6–1.2 per cent can be expected in combination with either metformin or a sulfonylurea.

Non-sulfonylurea Insulin Secretagogue

Repaglinide is a benzoic acid derivative of the meglitinides class which targets postprandial hyperglycemia. It is predominantly metabolized in the liver to inactive metabolites and is safe in mild to moderate renal impairment. It has a rapid onset of action and a relatively low risk of symptomatic hypoglycemia compared with sulfonylureas and has better postprandial glucose profiles. Tablets can be missed if meals are not taken, introducing a degree of `flexibility' in its use. It has been used effectively in combination with metformin and with glitazones (where license permits). It is recommended to start with 0.5mg at the start of each meal for subjects on diet, and 1.0 mg for patients transferring from other oral agents; up to 4 mg for each meal can be used. Nateglinide is a recent meglitinide that has a faster and shorter duration of insulin secretary activity than does Repaglinide.

Insulin

Insulin use in older people plays an increasingly important role in the management of diabetes. Recent improvements in the organization of care between hospital and primary care, together with the developing educational and diabetes care roles of diabetes specialist nurses and general practice nurses, have increased the availability and safety of insulin for older people with diabetes. Its main indications are in the treatment of type 1 diabetes at diagnosis, and in type 2 diabetes where metabolic targets have not been achieved with diet, exercise, and oral agents; other indications include its use in acute myocardial infarction, acute stroke, hyperglycemic coma, and major surgery. Its main disadvantage is hypoglycemia, although in the UKPDS less than 2 per cent subjects treated with insulin had a major episode of hypoglycemia. Few visual aids are available to assist those with poor vision in administering insulin, although some insulin pens have audible clicks for counting. Benefits of insulin include improvements in well-being (and possibly quality of life) and cognitive function in part due to improvements in glycemic control. However, these are not universal findings and treatment satisfaction may be lower in insulin-treated patients, suggesting that there is often a 'trade-off' between intensified control and quality of life – two important diabetes outcomes.

Practice-orientated Guidelines for Insulin Treatment in Older People

Once-daily insulin	*Twice daily insulin*	*Basal/bolus insulin*	*Insulin plus oral agent*
Frail subjects very old (>80 years) Symptomatic control	Preferred if good glycemic control suitable for type I diabetes	Well motivated individuals. Can reduce micro vascularcomplications	If glycemic control is unsatisfactory with oral agents alone.
Single injection Can be given by carer or district nurse	Low risk of hypoglycemia. Easily managed by most older diabetic people	Enables tight control for acute illness in hospital. Flexible meal times	Limits weight gain by reducing total daily insulin
Control usually poor Hypoglycemia common	Normoglycemia difficult to achieve fixed meal times reduce flexibility Expensive	Frequent monitoring required in avoiding hypoglycemia.	May delay conversion to insulin in thin or type 1 patients.

5 Arthritis

I.S. Gambhir

Epidemiology

Rheumatic problems are common in the elderly. Arthritis and musculoskeletal diseases are two of the most prevalent chronic conditions among elderly people. National Centre for Health Statistics (USA) observed that arthritis is the most common health condition affecting Americans over 50 years. Forty-nine per cent of the US population aged 65 to 74 years and 54 per cent persons over age 75 years have arthritis.[1]

Arthritis is the most common cause of disability in persons over 75 years.[2] The extent of arthritis related disabilities increases with ageing, as is shown by the longitudinal study data.[3] Arthritis (including Rheumatism) is one of most common causes of loss of mobility, and confinement in bed or in house.

Pain and limitations in movements can restrict the independence of elderly people by impairing activities of daily living (ADL). A hospital survey in London showed that 76 per cent of patients had peripheral arthritis and in 48 per cent arthritis directly contributed to functional disability.[4] According to National Health Survey, elderly persons with arthritis, living in the community, represent 70 per cent of the population with one or more limitations in physical activity and represent two-third of persons with an ADL impairment of five or more. They were 2–5 times more likely to die and five times more likely to be interned in nursing home in comparison to those without limitations.[5] Thus arthritis and musculoskeletal diseases in elderly significantly contribute to morbidity and mortality.

In a study of the rural living elderly in India,[6] 45 per cent of study subjects (n=215) had disabilities; out of these 88 per cent had locomotor problems. Almost all arthropathies have a high prevalence in old age. Several features of old age have a bearing on the pathogenesis of arthritis, such as decreased sex hormones, accumulation of free radical induced damages, degenerative changes in cartilage, loss of bone, muscle mass and immunosenescence. But arthropathies are active disorders with genetic and environmental factors. The ageing processes potentiate these or the cumulative effects of multiple processes are seen over years with ageing.[7]

Rheumatological problems in elderly people may have the following profiles:

(a) Some rheumatic conditions like osteoarthritis show a high prevalence in the elderly.
(b) Some rheumatic conditions like polymyalgia rheumatica and temporal arteritis occur exclusively in the elderly.
(c) Many rheumatological conditions like rheumatoid arthritis and gout occur both in young age and in elderly people.
(d) Many rheumatological conditions begin in young people, but because of their benign course and chronicity they often add to a high prevalence of rheumatoid arthritis and SLE in elderly patients.
(e) Association of non-rheumatological conditions like neoplasm with vasculitis and dermatomyositis.
(f) Iatrogenic disease like drug induced SLE and hypersensitivity angitis.

The common rheumatological problems in the elderly are described in Table 5.1:

Table 5.1 ***The Common Rheumatological Problems in the Elderly***

Condition	*Probable Pathogenesis*
Osteoarthritis	Degenerative arthritis
a. Rheumatoid arthritis	Inflammatory synovitis
b. Gout	
c. Crystal induced arthropathy (Pseudogout)	
Septic arthritis, tubercular	Infections
Polymyalgia rheumatica, Temporal arteritis	Vasculitis and connective tissue disease
Rotor cuff shoulder lesions, frozen shoulder	Vasculitis and connective tissue disease
Back Pain	Multiple causes may co-exist

Osteoarthiritis

Ageing is the most common risk factor for osteoarthritis (OA)[8] but an ageing joint differs from a joint afflicted by osteoarthritis (OA). In ageing joints the composition of proteoglycan changes and the water content of cartilage is diminished whereas in a joint affected by OA, the dominant feature is cartilage loss. The water content of cartilage is increased and inflammatory mediators suppress proteoglycan and collagen synthesis while degrading them.

Osteoarthritis (OA) is a heterogenous condition with a variety of causes and patterns of expression and is also termed as joint failure. The prevalence of OA rises with age, in Europe and North America the prevalence rises from under 1 per cent in below 35 years age group to over 30 per cent in 75 years or above age group.[9–10] Primary OA has on overall prevalence of 1.89 per cent in Indian population.[11]

Radiological evidence of osteoarthritis exceeds symptomatic OA. In 869 patients evaluated in the Framingham osteoarthritis study,[12] knee OA was 1.7 times more common in women, among women 2 per cent per year developed radiographic evidence of knee OA, 1 per cent per year developed symptomatic knee OA and 4 per cent experienced progression of knee OA.

Pathogenesis

Osteoarthritis is the result of hyaline cartilage degeneration exceeding regeneration. OA is a final common pathway of various causes of accelerated degeneration. Biomechanical factors like static load and prolonged cyclic loads inhibit synthesis of prostaglandins (PG) and proteins. OA develops in either of the two settings (a) Excessive loading of a joint with normal biomaterial properties of cartilage. This accounts for the high prevalence of OA at specific sites related to vocational or avocational overloading. (b) Inferior biomaterial quality of articular cartilage with normal loads. Clinical conditions that reduce the ability of cartilage to reform are associated with development of OA, e.g., in osteopetrosis, stiffness of the subchondral trabeculae occurs, and in onchronosis, accumulated homogentisic acid polymers stiffen cartilage. In both these conditions OA usually appears by 40 years.

The primary changes in OA begin in cartilage. Articular cartilage is composed of proteoglycan and collagen. There are irreversible changes in arrangement and size of collagen fibres, disrupting collagen network of the cartilage matrix. There is strong evidence that matrix metalloproteinases (MMPs) account for the major loss of cartilage matrix, along with plasmin and cathepsin. Synthesis or secretion of these MMPs by chondrocytes and other substances may be stimulated by IL-1, Nitric Oxide (NO), TNF or other factors like mechanical stimuli. TIMP and PAI-1 stabilize the system by inhibiting MMPs. IGF-1 and TGF β are supposed to be involved in the repair process through prostaglandins (Figure 5.1).

Figure 5.1 ***Factors Causing Articular Hyaline Cartilage Degeneration and Repair.***

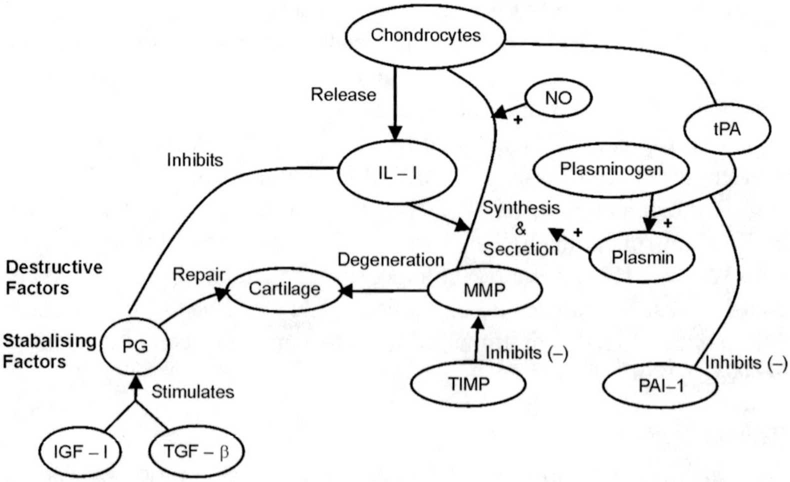

In OA cartilage, chondrocytes are active metabolically, and by dividing replicate. In the initial stage, in response to shear stress or other factors there may be increased biosynthetic activity with increased prostaglandins (PG) synthesis and thickening of cartilage. These compensatory mechanisms eventually fail in most cases with decline of PG synthesis, loss of cartilage and joint failure.

Abbreviations: IL-1 = Interleukin-1, MMP = Matrix metalloproteinases, PG = Prostaglandins, IGF-1 = Insulin growth factor-1, TGF-1 = Tissue growth factor-1, PAI-1 = Plasminogen activator inhibitor-1, tPA = Tissue plasminogen activator, TIMP = Tissue inhibitors of MMPs, (+) Stimulation, (–) Inhibition.

Cartilage in different joints respond in different ways to mechanical stress and exposure to cytokines and this accounts for the lower incidence of OA in some joints than others, e.g., ankle vs knee.

Pathology

The cardinal feature of OA is progressive loss of articular hyaline cartilage with fibrillation of cartilage surface as the earliest changes. Chondrocytes replicate to form clusters; areas of fibro cartilage repair develop and finally cartilage becomes hypo-cellular and thins out. Besides cartilage, subchondral bone, synovium, meniscus, ligaments all are involved. There is a remodeling of the subchondral bone, leading to bony sclerosis and growth of the cartilage and bone at joint margins lead to osteophytes. There is a thickening of joint capsule and chronic synovitis.

Subchondral bone is also involved in the pathogenesis, initiation and progression of OA; characterized by increased local bone turnover, decreased bone mineral content and stiffness, decreased trabecular numbers are seen in subchondral bone with OA as compared with trabecular normal bone.[13]

Classification of OA (Mankin et al.)[14]

(1) *Primary OA (Idiopathic):* is the most common form.
It is further classified into the following:

(i) Localized OA

(a) Hands – Nodal/Generalized OA
(b) Knee – Medial tibiofemoral, Lateral tibiofemoral, Patello-femoral
(c) Hip – Eccentric, Concentric, Diffuse
(d) Spine – Apophyseal, Intervertebral, Spondylosis, Ligamentous

(a) *Nodal or generalized HAND OA:* is characterized by involvement of distal interphalangeal joints (DIPs) and to a lesser extent proximal interphalangeal joints (PIPs), Heberdens nodes (due to bony enlargement of DIPs), Bouchard's nodes (due to bony enlargement of PIPs) and familial clustering. It is more common in females and is the best recognized subset.
(b) *The knee is the most common form of localized OA:* the knee joint may be the only joint involved; often bilateral, obesity, knee bending, female sex and age are risk factors.
(c) *Hip OA* is uncommon in India.
(d) *Spine:* It involves apophyseal joint, intervertebral disc. Intervertebral disc generation and osteophytes formation is common in cervical and lumber spine, the areas with maximum spinal motions.

Diffuse intraosseous skeletal hyperostosis (DISH) is characterized by calcification along anterior longitudinal ligaments and disc margins. OPLL is ossification of posterior longitudinal ligament. Both these are considered variables of OA.

(ii) *Generalized OA* is characterized by the involvement of more than three joints (i) Small peripheral joints (ii) Large central joints (axial) (iii) Mixed and spine.

(iii) *Erosive OA:* Marked by florid inflammation and erosive changes which lead to deformities and ankylosis. Usually interphalangeal joints (IPs) and hands are involved. Up to 15 per cent may later evolve into rheumatoid arthritis.

(2) Secondary Osteoarthritis

1. Post surgery – Menisectomy
2. Metabolic – Gout, Pseudo gout, Onchronosis
3. Associated with rheumatoid arthritis
4. Charcot joints
5. Intra-articular steroids
6. Hemophilic joints
7. Endocrine – DM, Acromegaly, Hyperparathyroidism, hypo or hyperthyroidism

Secondary osteoarthritis (OA) is characterized by (i) early onset <45 years of age, (ii) atypical sites, and (iii) polyarticular chondrocalcinosis.

Risk Factors for Primary Idiopathic OA

Risk factors for primary idiopathic OA are shown in Box 1.

Box 1 ***Risk Factors for Primary OA***

1. Increasing age
2. Female sex
3. Genetics
4. Obesity
5. Trauma, occupation and sports

Age: is the most important of risk factors. In a radiographic survey of women < 45 years only 2 per cent had OA, the prevalence was 30 per cent in the age group 45–65 years and 68 per cent in 65 years and above. In males the figures were similar but somewhat lower.[15] The prevalence of symptomatic OA increased from 7.0 per cent in the 63–69 years age group to over 11.2 per cent in the over 80 years of age group in the Framingham cohort. Besides incidence, the severity of OA also increased with age (grade 3/4 changes from 11.5 per cent in 60s to 19.4 per cent in 80s).[16]

Sex: Females have greater incidence of knee and hand OA, more severe OA and greater symptoms.[17] Males have greater incidence of hip OA (in > 55 years age group), but when all joints OA is taken together, no significant sex difference is discernible.

Race: There may be racial differences in pattern of joint involvements (for e.g., Indians have high prevalence of knee OA but low prevalence of hip or hand OA). These differences may be genetic or environmental; this aspect is not well studied. No mutations have been identified in primary idiopathic OA, though twin studies have shown 65 per cent concordance for developing OA.[18] Certain familial OA have been found to have point mutations in gene coding for collagen-II (COL 2A1). Heberden's nodes are inherited in women in autosomal dominant form and in men in autosomal recessive form.

Obesity: Obesity has a strong association with knee and hand OA but not hip OA.[19] In Framingham study, obese women, overweight women and obese men, all had an increased risk of developing OA over 25 years (relative risk 2.07, 1.44 and 1.51 respectively) while overweight men did not have an increased risk (relative risk 1).[16] Obese patients are more likely to have a progressive disease.[20] A weight reduction of 5 kg decreases the risk of symptomatic OA in obese patient by 50 per cent.

Joint trauma and repetitive joint uses: are also significant risk factors for OA,[21] e.g., menisectomy is associated with a high risk for secondary OA. Similarly, previous history of knee injury increased the risk of radiographic OA three-fold in males and two-fold in females, and increased the risk of symptomatic OA significantly.[16] Damage to articular cartilage may occur at the time of injury or subsequently with the use of a joint. Even the normal cartilage in an affected joint may degenerate, if the joint is unstable. Prior vocational or avocational overload of the joint (repetitive joint use) may determine the pattern of joint involvement, e.g., farmers have OA hip,[22] ankle OA is most common in ballet dancers, elbow OA in baseball players and metacarpophalangeal joint OA in prize fighters. However, no convincing data is available describing an association between nonprofessional athletic or sport activities and OA. Chondrocalcinosis imparted a small but significant risk factor for OA knee.

Clinical features of OA: Some joints are more commonly involved in primary idiopathic OA and some are rarely involved (Box 2). OA is characterized by joint pain, stiffness, and functional disability.

Box 2 ***Joint Involvement Pattern in Primary OA***

Commonly involved	*Uncommon*	*Rare*
Knee	Hip Joint	Elbow
Spine (Apophyseal)	Acromioclavicular	Ankle
Hand (PIP, DIP and	Sternoclavicular	Carpal
Ist CMC Joint)		Glenohumoral
		Intertarsal

Symptoms

Joint pain: in OA is a deep ache, poorly localized to involved joint, aggravated by joint use and relieved by rest initially but later on with disease progression, it may become persistent. Joint pain arises from other joint structures like synovium, joint capsule, and cartilage being aneural. Muscle spasm may contribute to pain.

Stiffness: May be morning stiffness lasting less than 30 minutes, or more characteristically may come after inactivity when it is frequently termed "gelling". Stiffness may refer to difficulty in initiating movements, problem in completing a full range of movement or the ache or pain of joint on movement. Loss of movement or joint instability, a sudden feeling of the joint giving way may be other complaints.

Signs: Physical examination may be normal in early OA, with the progression of disease there may be bony or soft tissue swellings.

Swellings: Most characteristic bony swellings are Heberden's and Bouchard's nodes of hand OA. Synovial effusion occurs in some cases especially in knee OA, usually it is not large. Palpation may reveal tenderness and/or warmth over the affected joint; but usually very mild and uncommon and are likely to be due to micro crystal deposition.

Crepitus is common and present in 90 per cent of knee OA. It results from cartilage loss and joint surface irregularity.

Joint motion: Restriction of range of motion (ROM) is due to capsular contraction, decreased joint space, muscle spasm, osteophytes and loose bodies. There may be joint instability and joint deformity in advanced OA due to destruction of cartilage and other joint structures. Periarticular muscle atrophy may be due to disease or reflex inhibition of muscle contraction. The clinical features of OA at specific joint sites are given in Table 5.2.

Table 5.2 ***Clinical Features of OA at Specific Joint Site***

Knee	*Spine*	*Hands*	*Hip*
There may be tenderness/bony swelling (osteophytes) pain and crepitus is present on movement of joint. Varus/valgus deformity in the case of tibio-femoral OA and shrug sign in patelofemoral OA may be present weakness or atrophy of quadriceps.	Diagnosis is reserved for patients with involvement of apophysea joints, there is localized pain and stiffness, due to associated spondylosis, or sublaxation of apophyseal joint. There may be radicular pain and motor weakness.	Heberden's and Bouchard's nodes are characteristic. There may be a dorsal cyst at the insertion of digital extensor tendons into the base of the distal phalanx. Thumb base involvement presents as swelling, tenderness and crepitus on movement. There is a loss of motion and strength. Osteophytes leads to a "squared" appearance.	Pain is generally referred to inguinal area, but may be referred to the buttock, proximal thigh or even the knee. Internal rotation is the first to be affected followed by extension, adduction and flexion.

Natural course: OA is chronic and irreversible but course is variable. In long-term studies one-third to two-third OA may progress, the rest may remain stable but improvements are rare. Symptomatic OA may progress, improve or remain stable. Symptoms do not correlate well with radiological progression.[20,23] Patients with multiple joints OA have more rapid progression than single joint OA; advance age[24] and obesity[22] may be risk factors for the progression of OA. Cushnhaan & Dieppe[25] found a strong relationship between age and the number of joints involved. Inflammatory OA and destructive OA disease, mostly in elderly women forms a subset with radio graphic findings of rapid severe destruction of the joint mimicking RA, Sepsis. It mainly affects shoulders, knees and hips. Joint destruction is complete within 1–2 years.[26]

Investigations

Radiology: In early OA, radiographs may be normal but a decrease in joint space (JS) is evident with loss of cartilage. Other characteristic findings are osteophytes, subchondral bone sclerosis and subchondral cysts. None of the radiographic findings are diagnostic in isolation, although for knee OA, tibiofemoral joint space narrowing has been considered a radiographic surrogate for articular cartilage thinning, though it alone does not accurately indicate the status of articular cartilage in early OA. Osteophytosis may be due to ageing and not OA. In certain joints such as knees, films should be obtained in weight bearing positions to assess degree of joint space narrowing. The common radiographic grading system of OA is Kellgren and Lawrence scale. There is often great disparity between radiographic features of OA, clinical symptoms and functional ability in primary OA. While >90 per cent patients over 40 years have some radiographic features of OA in weight-bearing joints, only 30 per cent are symptomatic.

Role of arthroscopy is restricted to the removal of loose bodies. MRI and USG are not recommended for routine clinical use for diagnosis of OA or for monitoring of progression of OA

Lab Investigations: No lab studies are diagnostic in primary OA though they may help to identity secondary causes of OA. In primary OA, ESR, CRP, blood counts, serum chemistry and urinalysis are normal. Synovial fluid analysis reveals mild leucocytosis (<2000 white blood cells per ml) with predominance of mononuclear cells. Synovial fluid analysis is crucial to rule out other conditions especially crystal induced arthropathy, gout or septic arthritis. Molecular markers like keratan sulfate, pyrindinoline, chondroitin sulfate, neoepitope, collagen II-C peptide, chondroitin 6 sulphate/4 sulphate ratio, osteocalcin and hyauluronic acid may be detected in increased amounts in serum, urine and synovial fluids in OA.[27] None of these have found clinical usefulness in diagnosis or monitoring of OA progression.

Diagnosis: Although the diagnosis of established OA with typical clinical and radiological features is usually straight forward, joint pain with radiographic evidence of OA does not necessarily mean symptomatic OA due to a high prevalence of asymptomatic radiographic changes. Joint pain in such cases may be due to soft tissue rheumatism (e.g., Anserine bursitis at knee joint), referral pain from hip disease, other arthropathies (crystal induced, septic), radiculopathy, entrapment neuropathy, vascular disease (intermittent claudication) etc. Differentiation from rheumatoid arthritis (RA) is usually easy due to the pattern of joint involvement, constitutional symptoms and lab findings of inflammation in RA. Inflammatory OA with destructive disease (erosive arthritis), seen more commonly in elderly females, is especially problematic. The radiographic changes may mimic septic arthritis, rheumatoid and sero-negative arthritis. There is rapid progression of pain and disability leading to complete joint destruction in 1–2 years. The condition may affect shoulders, knees and hips.

Difficulties also arise in early OA when physical and radiological features may be normal and clinical presentation may be atypical. For epidemiological and research purposes, the American Rheumatism Association (ARA) has proposed following diagnostic criteria for OA in different joints given in Tables 5.3[28], 5.4[29], and 5.5[30].

Table 5.3 ***Knee Osteoarthritis – Clinical and Radiological Classification Criteria***

Traditional Format	*Classification Tree Format*
Knee pain Osteophytes Plus One of three: Age >50 years Stiffness < 30 minutes Crepitus	Knee pain and Osteophytes or Knee pain and age = 40 years and morning stiffness = 30 minutes in duration and crepitus on motion

Altman et al. 1986, Arthritis Rheum 29:1039–1049.

Table 5.4 ***Osteoarthritis of the Hip-Classification Criteria Traditional Format***

Hip pain
At least two of the following:
ESR Westergreen <20mm/hr
Radiographic femoral or acetabular osteophytes
Radiographic joint space narrowing (superior, axial, and/or medial)

89 per cent sensitive, 91 per cent specific; Altman et al., 1991, Arthritis Rheum 34:505–514.

Table 5.5 ***Osteoarthritis of the Hand – Classification Criteria: Traditional Format***

Hand pain, aching, or stiffness
Three or four of the following
Hard tissue enlargement of 2 or more of 10 selected joints*
Hard tissue enlargement of 2 or more DIP joints
Less than 3 swollen MCP joints
Deformity of at least one of the 10 selected joints

*10 selected joints are 2nd and 3rd DIP joints, 2nd and 3rd PIP joints, and 1st carpometacarpal joint.

94 per cent sensitive, 87 per cent specific; Altman et al. 1990, Arthritis Rheum 30: 1601–1610

These clinical criteria developed for diagnosing OA, have been criticized for lacking age and sex matched controls, using osteophytes as a feature of OA, for circular justification and inadequate validation.[31]

Treatment of OA: There is no curative treatment for OA at present. The present treatment modalities are aimed at reducing pain, maintaining mobility, minimizing disability with minimum side effects. The comprehensive approach in treatment of OA involves non-pharmacological, pharmacological and surgical interventions. The American College of Rheumatology (ACR) guidelines for managing OA knee and hip are given in Tables 5.6 and 5.7.[32,33]

Table 5.6 ***Non-Pharmacological Therapy in Osteoarthritis (ACR Guidelines)***

Patient education
Self management programmes (e.g., Arthritis self-help course)
Health professional social support via telephone contact
Weight loss (if overweight)
Physical therapy
Range of motion exercises
Strengthening exercises
(Quadriceps exercises in knee)
Assistive devices for ambulation
Occupational therapy
Joint protection and energy conservation
Assistive devices for activities of daily living (ADLs) and instrumental activities of daily (IADLs)
Aerobic exercise programmes (aquatic for hip)

Table 5.7 ***Medical Management of Symptomatic Osteoarthritis of the Hip and Knee***

Non-pharmacologic therapy
If effusion present, consider aspiration and injection of intra-articular steroids (e.g., triamcinolone hexacetonide)
Acetaminophen (up to 1gm qid) for pain and symptom control
If necessary, add topical capsaicin cream
If response inadequate, use alternative analgesic, low dose ibuprofen (up to 400mg qid) or non-acetylated salicylates
If response inadequate, use full-dose non-steroidal anti-inflammatory drug (with misoprostol if patient has risk factors for UGI bleeding or ulcer disease)
If response inadequate and surgery is contraindicated, consider referral for joint lavage and/or arthroscopic debridement
If response inadequate, and surgery is not contraindicated, consider referral for joint surgery (osteotomy, total joint arthroplasty)
These measures are applicable for knee joint only.

Modified from Hochberg et al., 1995.

Non-Pharmacological Treatment

Patient Education: Emphasis should be placed upon joint protection like avoidance of poor postures, limitation of joint loading. Patient with knee or hip OA should avoid long standing, kneeling and squatting, by changing toilet seats, avoiding stair climbing, and using walking sticks. Occupational therapists can play an important role in teaching patients joint protection techniques and general coping strategies, using aids, assistive devices and gadgets. Patient education about the disease process and its management include providing patients with educational materials and support for self-management.

Reduction in Joint Loading: In patients with medial compartment knee OA, a wedged insole may decrease joint pain due to a decrease in joint loading. A polypropylene mesh insole is inexpensive and cost effective. Loss of weight in obese patients is highly desired to reduce joint loading. Though complete immobilization of the painful joint is rarely required, except in hand OA, rest periods during the day may be beneficial. For painful DIP joints OA, interfering with hand function, a suitable thermoplastic splint blocking flexion will improve muscle spasm, reduce pain and improve overall hand function. However rigid immobilization is not an acceptable long-term option for PIPs as it limits hand function and causes shortening of collateral ligaments. In patients with unilateral OA knee or hip, a cane held in opposite hand may reduce joint pain. Bilateral disease may necessitate use of crutches or a walker.

Patellar Taping: In patellofemoral compartment OA of the knee, severe pain may occur with kneeling, climbing stairs or squatting. Medial taping of patella can reduce pain in such cases to a great extent. The procedure is simple, inexpensive and can be learned by the patient, who can tape it at home when required. On a long-term basis, this may be followed by isometric exercises of vastus medialis obliqus component of quadriceps to realign patella.

Exercise: is needed for treatment of OA as well as for general health. Physical therapy is the measure most commonly employed to optimize joint biomechanics. Disuse of the joint due to pain leads to periarticular muscle atrophy, which further adds to the destruction of articular cartilage, thus perpetuating a vicious cycle. In knee OA patients, strengthening of the periarticular muscles may result in a decrease of joint pain equivalent to NSAIDs within weeks. Though most of the available information is about the muscle strengthening aspect of exercises, the therapeutic benefits go far beyond. With proper patient education, compliance is excellent; there is overall feeling of well-being; a reduction in joint pain, anxiety, depression and disability; and an increase in lower extremity strength, endurance and functional ability. Patients performing range of motion exercises as compared to isometric exercises for muscle strengthening did not have significant improvement in joint pain or strength. Aerobic capacity of men with severe OA is 30 per cent less than age matched normal controls without OA. Aerobic exercises are necessary for cardiovascular fitness in the elderly and this can be achieved even in elderly patients with OA. Patients with lower extremity OA, who are able to exercise at least 3 days a week with 70–85 per cent of predicted maximal heart rate, are able to improve their cardiovascular fitness without exacerbating their joint pain or using NSAIDs. Aerobic exercises have been shown to be beneficial in OA in improving fitness and self-dependence.[34] Normal movements and loading of joints maintain the integrity of the affected joint and facilitate repair of the damaged cartilage. Hence, patients should be advised to remain active within individual limitations during the quiescent phase of OA. During inflammation with significant joint pain, overstress with exercise should be avoided. A comprehensive rest-exercise programme is recommended, with the rationale that activity aids repair and rest allows rehydration of cartilage.

Measures to Reduce Pain

Application of heat may reduce pain and stiffness; most convenient is a hot shower or bath. Occasionally better analgesia is achieved with ice than heat in acutely inflamed joints. Ultrasound and massage are other modalities of treatment to relieve pain, muscle spasm and decrease stiffness of joint.

Pharmacological treatment: It may be grouped according to function.

(A) *For Pain Relief:* Analgesia may be achieved by acetaminophen (APAP), nonselective NSAIDs (Ibuprofen, Diclofenac, Naproxen), Cox-2 inhibitors (Valdecoxib, Celecoxib, Rofecoxib), opoid agonists (Codeine or Tramadol).

Acetaminophen (APAP): are currently first line drug for relief of pain especially in elderly, due to its moderate effective analgesia with good safety profile. The usual dose of APAP is 4gm/day given 3–4 times. NSAIDs are added only if analgesia is not adequate. Studies have shown APAP to be as effective as NSAIDs.[22] Majority of large sized clinical trials, comparing nonselective NSAIDs with APAP, have shown only small effect sizes, with the distributions of reduction of pain overlapping in more than 80 per cent patients.[35] In nearly 50 per cent patients, APAP was judged by patients to be as good as NSAIDs, with the percentage of those preferring APAP increasing with age.[36] Similar results have been seen in a recent double blind crossover trial.[37]

Non-selective NSAIDs

The magnitude of improvement with NSAIDs is modest as compared to placebo, with 30 per cent relief in pain and 15 per cent in function.[38–39] The use of nonselective NSAIDs has been a cause of concern particularly in elderly patients due to adverse drug reactions, involving GI tract, renal, hepatic, CNS, cardiovascular and haemorrhage. There is a four-times greater risk of GI events (Peptic ulcer, GI Hgg. Perforation and death) in an elderly NSAIDs user. In the 65 years and above age group, 30 per cent of hospitalization and deaths related to peptic ulcer disease are attributed to NSAIDs.[15] Some NSAIDs like Aspirin and indomethacin have been implicated in cartilage destruction and shall be avoided.

Selective NSAIDs (Cox-2 inhibitors)

Cox-2 inhibitors (Coxib) have no greater efficacy than nonselective NSAIDs.[40–41] In VACT study Celecoxib at 200mg/day was not significantly more efficacious than APAPs.[42] Although Rofecoxib at 25mg/day was more effective, the VIGOR study underlined a four-fold rise in acute MI among patients treated with Rofecoxib as compared to patients treated with Naproxen[43]; increased vulnerability has also been noted with Celecoxib and may be a class effect. Furthermore retention of salt and water associated with Cox-2 inhibitors may lead to edema, hypertension, CHF, and reduction of the efficacy of antihypertensive drugs. Although serious GI side effects (GI bleeding, peptic ulcer) decreased by 50–60 per cent with Rofecoxib as compared to non selective NSAID Naproxen in the VIGOR trial, a large GI safety study of Celecoxib (Class trial)[44] is less clear and concomitant use of low dose of aspirin in elderly mitigate any GI protective effect of Celecoxib. The incidence of symptomatic ulcers and potentially fatal ulcer complications (i.e., haemorrhage, perforation) is about 2–5 per cent a year in patients taking non-selective NSAIDs[45–46], with the risk being greater in patients with advanced age, co-morbidities, history of peptic ulcer disease or upper GI bleed and anticoagulant therapy. The adverse renal, hepatic, CNS and haematological side effect profile of nonselective

NSAIDs is similar to Cox-2 inhibitors and so is the adverse effect on fracture healing with both. Thus, though Cox-2 inhibitors (Coxibs) have a GI safety advantage over nonselective NSAIDs, the increased risk of vascular thrombosis and Acute MI, results in unacceptable increase in mortality and morbidity, which is a significant disadvantage especially in the elderly, hence use of Coxibs is not recommended.

Opoid Agonists: Codeine has been used for its analgesic effect in OA for longtime for acute flare up. Codeine in doses of 60mg is not more effective than APAP; hence a combination is preferred for treating moderate or moderately severe OA. Chronic use of codeine or propoxyphene has been limited because of its side effects profile, e.g., nausea, vomiting, constipation urinary retention, respiratory depression, mental confusion and drowsiness. These drugs increase the risk of fall and hip fractures by 60 per cent[15] in addition to being addictive. Tramadol, a centrally acting analgesic with ì. opioid activity have opioid and non-opioid analgesic effects, which are synergistic. The analgesic effect is comparable to NSAID[47] Ibuprofen but has no side effects on GI, renal or platelets as it does not inhibit prostaglandins. Tolerance and dependence is uncommon and hence, it is not a scheduled drug. The efficacy and safety profile of Tramadol is comparable to codeine; which is much cheaper, though lesser constipation is reported with tramadol. Its analgesic effect however, is not greater than APAP.A combination of Tramadol in low doses (37.5 mg) with APAP is comparable to an APAP and codeine combination for acute flair of OA. With chronic use, lower side effects have been observed with tramadol if the drug is started at 25 mg and slowly increased, e.g., "start low and go slow" approach. However, due to inhibition of reuptake of both norepinephrine and serotonin, concomitant use of TCA and SSRIs in the elderly may cause seizures, which may occur even when tramadol is used alone, though with lesser frequency.

Topical Analgesics: for OA are useful adjuncts to other analgesics in moderate to severe OA and may be useful alone in mild OA. A Rubefacients application may work by local heat generation. Capsaicin works by depletion of substance P in sensory nerve endings by causing local irritation.

Disease Modifying Agents

Glucosamine and Chondroitin Sulphate: Several studies have shown that glucosamine has a greater efficacy than a placebo, is comparable to NSAIDs in patients with knee OA, and has better safety profile[48]. In a meta-analysis of randomized, double blind, placebo controlled studies of glucosamine and chondroitin sulphate, moderate symptomatic benefit was shown by both agents relative to placebo; however the effect size of both agents was lower in trials with better study designs. Moreover, in three recent randomized double blind trials, glucosamine was no more effective than placebo. The chondroprotective effect of glucosamine, chondroitin sulphate or their combination in knee osteoarthritis is under investigation and not yet settled.

MMPs Inhibitors: The metalloproteinases (MMPs) have been shown to play a central role in cartilage degeneration. Tetracycline is one potent inhibitor of MMPs. Treatment of OA knee in obese women patients with Doxycycline, as compared to placebo, significantly reduced follow up visits due to pain and caused decrease in joint space narrowing.[49] Chemically modified Tetracyclines (CMTs) without antibacterial action but with inhibitors in MMPs seems to be promising disease modifying agents. Patients presenting with significant inflammation with demonstrable CPPD crystals have better symptomatic relief with Colchicine which may have a disease modifying role.

Bisphosphonates

Osteoporosis was long considered to be protective for osteoarthritis (OA); but recent evidence has suggested a role of subchondral bones in both irritation and progression of OA. A recent cross sectional study has observed an association between antiresorptive treatments (oestrogen and bisphosphanate) and improvement in knee OA symptoms. Treatment of knee OA with risedronate 15 mg resulted in a consistent improvement in WOMAC Score as compared to placebo and showed a decrease in joint space narrowing.[50] However, similar improvements with risedronate was not seen in OA patients in a multicentric study.[51]

Invasive Procedures

(a) *Intra-Articular Steroids:* Intra or Peri-articular injection of a depot glucocorticoid preparation provide marked symptomatic relief in severe OA, lasting weeks or months. Studies in animal models have suggested cartilage damage with glucocorticoids, and in humans frequent injections of large amount of steroids have been associated with joint breakdown, hence the use of intra-articular injections should not exceed 3–4 times in a given joint and shall not be repeated before 4–6 months. Systemic steroids have no place in treatment of OA.

(b) *Intra-Articular Hyaluron (IA-HA):* IA-HA has been used in patients not responding to APAP, NSAIDs or non pharmacological therapy. Though the mechanism is unclear, viscosupplementation is claimed as the basis for clinical improvement, which is supposed to last for several months. However, IA-HA was found to increase viscosity of synovial fluid only transiently.[52] Diepe et al. in an analysis of 11 clinical trials of IA-HA found the pooled effect size to be 0.48 (with 95% CI of 0.72–0.23). These studies show no reduction in NSAIDs use. Recent studies have failed to show any significant benefit of IA-HA over saline injection or degraded HA (with markedly reduced viscoelasticity).[54–55]

(c) *Tidal Irrigation:* Irrigation of the knee joint by a large bore needle flushes out fibrin, small cartilage fragments and other debris, but a randomized controlled clinical trial has shown it to be no better than placebo.[15]

(d) *Chondroplasty:* or abrasion arthroplasty has not shown any efficacy in well controlled studies; the fibro cartilage that resurfaces on the abraded bone is inferior to normal hyaline cartilage and symptomatic relief and functional ability did not improve significantly. Autologous chondrocyte transplantation and mesenchymal stem cells are being experimented with for repair of focal chondral defects but without much success.

(e) *Arthroscopic Lavage and Debridement:* Arthroscopic removal in OA patients with loose bodies, and debridement in patients with disruption of meniscus or cartilage provides relief of symptoms like lock knee or other mechanical symptoms. However, it has no role in OA patients without mechanical symptoms.

Orthopedic Surgery

Charnley revolutionized joint replacement therapy in severe OA, not manageable by other means. Most OA patients with joint arthroplasty have significant clinical improvement in joint pain, function and quality of life.[56,57] Osteotomy, a conservative surgery, provides effective pain relief in moderately severe OA knee or hip by reducing peak dynamic load.

Management of Osteoarthritis

In the treatment of OA, non-pharmacological treatment is the foundation and most important, drug treatment plays a secondary role with individualization of treatment. For analgesic treatment, topical analgesia shall be given a fair trial, alone in mild OA or as an adjunct in moderate to severe OA. APAP shall be the first analgesic, it shall be given up to 4gms/day. In case of failure to obtain symptomatic relief within a reasonable time (2–3 weeks), nonselective NSAIDs shall be added in low doses or substituted for APAP. Lowest effective dose of NSAIDs shall be used (to avoid ADRs) and these may be prescribed on an "as needed basis" rather than as fixed doses. The dose of NSAIDs may be lowered during chronic stage. To avoid GI side effects in vulnerable group, a non selective NSAIDs may be added with a proton pump inhibitor which has been shown to prevent NSAIDs induced gastropathy. Coxibs are no longer recommended due to their side effect profile. Codeine or Tramadol may be added during acute flare ups. Glucosamine or chondroitin sulphate have failed to demonstrate any significant benefit so far and hence are not recommended. MMP inhibitors are still in the experimental phase. Systemic steroids have no role. The role of bisphosphonates is not clear. Intra-articular steroids may be used in severe OA with marked inflammation but sparingly for symptomatic relief. Intra-articular Hyaluron has not been proven better than placebo; nor has tidal irrigation of joint and chondroplasty. Arthroscopic removal of loose bodies has been useful in relief of mechanical symptoms of OA only. Osteotomy and joint arthroplasty has been effective in symptomatic relief and improving function of joint.

Crystal Induced Arthropathies

In this group two common problems in elderly people are gout and pseudogout.

Gout is due to deposition of monosodium urate monohydrate crystals (MSUM). In the elderly tophaceous or non tophaceous gout occurs due to an idiopathic decrease in urate secretion, a decrease in renal function or use of certain diuretics or drugs, the latter causes being the most common. The prevalence of gout increases with ageing and approaches 4 per cent in 50–74 years old. Most common joints first affected are metatarsophalangeal joint, metatarsals, ankle, knee, small joints of hands, wrist or elbow. Axial joints or large proximal joints are rarely involved, never as first site. The involved joint is acutely tender, red, hot and swollen, mimicking acute infection. Initially attacks are monoacrticular but subsequent attack may be polyarticular and associated with fever. The acute attacks are self-limiting lasting 1–2 weeks. Acute attacks may also manifest as bursitis, tenosynovitis or cellulitis. The asymptomatic period between attacks may range from within 1 year to several years. Over the course of a decade, with MSUM deposits, joint damage and chronic pain develop. In the elderly, gout is never primary but usually secondary, presenting more commonly as painful tophi, with hands more predominantly involved than feet.[58] Gout may develop in joints with primary OA, presenting a diagnostic riddle. Drugs like thiazide or loop diauretics (an use of >18 months), pyrazinamide, and low dose aspirin are associated with gout in elderly people. In the elderly on long-term diuretic therapy, the association of nodal generalized osteoarthritis is an important additional risk factor for developing gout.

Diagnosis is made by demonstrating urate crystals in synovial fluid. There is poor correlation between hyperuricemia (S. Uric acid >7.0mg/dl in elderly men and postmenopausal women) and acute gout; in up to 30 per cent the uric acid levels may be in normal range. The acute gout is due to acute crystallization of urate (MSUM) or from shedding of crystals in synovium as may occur with rapid decrease in serum uric acid levels. In the treatment of an acute attack, NSAIDs and colchicine are best avoided due to toxicity; instead aspiration of the joint and intra articular injection of steroids is more helpful. Long-term treatment consists of stopping any drugs causing hyperuricemia, lifestyle modifications, (high purine diet, beer, obesity management). Prolonged treatment for hyperuricemia is needed in the presence of tophi, associated renal disease, severe hyperuricemia, evidence of joint damage or recurrent attacks of gout. Allopurinol is the drug of choice, the usual dose is 100–300 mg/day; but in elderly people low dosages (100 mg or less) should be used; dosages should be further reduced in the presence of renal insufficiency. The sharp reduction of S. uric acid may dissolve MSUM crystals and may precipitate an attack of acute gout.

Calcium Pyrophosphate Dihydrate (CPPD) Crystal deposition: Hyaline and fibrocartilage of joints (chondrocalcinosis) increases with age. In the age group 65–75 years 10–15 per cent persons have evidence of CPPD. This increases to 30–60 per cent after age 85 years. There is a female preponderance and in the Framingham study covering the age group 63 to 93 years, the prevalence rate was 8 per cent.[59] The mean age of presentation is 65–75 years. Joints most commonly affected are knee (hyaline cartilage and menisci), wrist (triangular fibrocartilage) and symphysis pubis. CPPD deposition is usually sporadic but may be familial or associated with other metabolic diseases. There is a strong association and overlap with OA. In up to one-third of the elderly there is only x-ray evidence of CPPD deposition (chondrocalcinosis) in the meniscus of the knee, triangular ligament of the wrist and occasionally the cartilage of shoulder. In others it may present as acute synovitis (Pseudogout), subacute or chronic pyrophosphate arthritis.

Acute Pyrophosphate Arthritis (Pseudogout): Most common cause of monoarthritis in the elderly, the knee is the commonest site, followed by the wrist, shoulder, ankle and elbow. It may occur in the background of chronic pyrophosphate arthritis as an exacerabation or may be the first presentation in an asymptomatic CPPD. The classical presentation is acute synovitis of pseudogout, the typical attack develops with severe pain, stiffness and swelling maximal within 6–24 hrs of onset. Overlying erythema is common. There is a marked tenderness with large/tense effusion, warmth, restricted movement with stress pain (features of synovitis). Fever is common. The acute attacks are self-limiting but may take 1–3 weeks to resolve. Pseudogout has to be differentiated from septic arthritis or gout. There may be coexistance of sepsis and psedugout. Gout seldom involves the knee and is rare in >65 years without a history of primary disease or chronic diuretic therapy. Pseudogout may present as bursitis or tenderness as well.

Chronic Pyrophosphate Arthritis: More common in elderly women, it involves knee, wrists and shoulder joints. In the hand 2nd and 3rd MCP joints are most affected. Presentation is similar to OA i.e., chronic pain, early morning and inactivity stiffness; reduced movements and functional impairment. There is crepitus and bony swellings, effusions and soft tissue thickening. There may be recurrent acute attacks; monoarthritis or polyarthritis may be present. Due to inflammatory features, a distinction from RA is difficult at times, but the absence of extra-articular features, tenosynovitis and involvement of the large joints rather than the small joints is differentiating. In most patients there is a benign course and the majority show a stabilization of symptoms[60]. Occasionally there is a progressive severe destructive arthritis especially involving the knee, shoulders or hips, almost exclusively in elderly women, usually with severe night and rest pain and a poor outcome.[61]

Management

Aspiration of synovial fluid and identification of calcium pyrophosphate crystals on polarized microscopy is suggestive. Definite diagnosis of crystal induced arthritis can be made if ingested crystals are seen piercing through phogocytic cells. The fluid is usually turbid, and may be blood-stained with characteristic inflammatory features. Radiographs may show chondrocalcinosis in hyaline and/or fibrocartilage, occasionally in capsule or ligaments with osteoarthritis pattern of joint destruction and calcification. Absence of chondrocalcinosis does not rule out pseudogout. Acute pseudogout may cause raised ESR/CRP and leucocytes. Aspiration of synovial fluids in acute stage, and relief with analgesic and NSAIDs, greatly improves symptoms. Colchicine is effective but rarely used in severe polyarticular attack, as it is unresponsive to aspiration. Oral steroids may be used. However their efficacy is unproven. There is no specific therapy and treatment, along with general measures, is symptomatic.

Apatite Deposition Disease: Periarticular or articular deposition of hydroxyapatite (a component of bone) or carbonated apatites of calcium can cause periarthritis or arthritis.

Calcific deposition in the supraspinatus tendon is a common incidental radiographic findings (7% of adults). It occasionally results in severe acute inflammation of subacromial bursa through crystal shedding into and around bursa; less commonly periarticular sites around greater trochanter of hip, foot or hand may be involved. Radiographs show tendon calcification and aspirate from subacromial bursa shows calcium stained aggregates. In some patients there is acute synovitis. A rapidly destructive arthritis due to hydroxyapatite seen in elderly people, termed "Milwaukee shoulder syndrome" has been described.[62] Patients are usually of 70 years or more, mostly females (90%), with or without a history of chronic joint disease.[63] Radiographic presence of calcific periarticular or associated changes within a joint is seen. Aspiration microscopy showing presence of apatite crystals is suggestive. Asymptomatic individuals with apatite crystals deposition need no treatment. Acute attacks are managed with similar lenses of crystal induced synoritis. There is no specific treatment.

Rheumatoid Arthritis (RA)

The prevalence of RA increases with age, being more frequent in elderly women. It was rare before 45 years in males and 35 years in females. In the over 65 years age group its prevalence increased to 1.8 per cent in males and 4.9 per cent in females.[64] RA being a chronic disease may be carried over into the elderly age group or may be appearing for the first time (late onset RA). Healey et al. (1986)[65] describes RA in the elderly as an entity with 3 subsets. The classical RA in the elderly is one subset. Such patients constitute 4 per cent of elderly RA in India.[66] Late onset RA is another subset. A small number of patients have atypical onset which include intermittent episodes of arthritis termed palindromic rheumatism, polymyalgic and monoarticular onset. Palindromic arthritis is symptom complex rather than a disease and may evolve into RA.[67] It is characterized by transient synovial inflammation and involvement of different joints. Polymyalgic onset is marked by predominant shoulder girdle symptoms. In monoarticular onset knee joint is frequently involved. The cervical spine is a common site of involvement in elderly. A condition, remitting seronegative symmetrical synovitis with pitting edema, primary affecting elderly, has been observed in a small group. In Indian patients also clinical features are similar but with less morning stiffness and more deformities. Seropositively is frequent. Characteristic features of late onset RA are shown in Box 3.

Box 3 ***Showing Characteristic Features of Late Onset RA in the Elderly***

1. Sex incidence is equal.
2. Morning stiffness is severe and prolonged.
3. Onset is frequently acute.
4. Greater predilection for larger joints, shoulder joints affected in >50 per cent.
5. Deformities are less common, systemic symptoms are common and prognosis is favourable.
6. ESR is very high, and a rheumatoid factor is frequently present.
7. Radiological erosive changes are less frequent.

Course

The RA in elderly people is progressive in the majority (70%) with some fluctuations in severity. In others remissions are usually not long (>10%). In 5 per cent the RA may take a malignant course with severe extra-articular disease especially vasculitis.

Diagnosis

RA and OA are both common diseases in the elderly age group and may 2coexist; hence differentiation between RA and OA can be difficult (Box 4). Other conditions that can mimic RA include polymyalgia rheumatica, late onset SLE, crystal induced arthropathies.

Box 4 *Differentiation Between RA and OA.*

Symptoms	*OA*	*RA*
Joint stiffness	< 30 minutes	> 30 minutes
Arthritis	Pauci articular, asymmetric	Symmetric, distal polyarticular
Joint involvement	KJ, spine, hand- DIP, PIP	Wrist joints, MCP, MTP, PIP KJ, AJ.
Features of joint inflammation	Minimal	Present
Systemic features	Absent	Present
Investigation		
ESR, CRP	Normal	Raised
RA factor	Negative	Present
Synovial fluid	<2000 cells	> 3000 cells

ACR diagnostic criteria for RA holds true for the elderly also, though RA factor false positivity is higher. ESR is a good and cheap monitoring tool with significant correlations between high ESR and other disease activity measures and destructive RA[68] but mildly elevated ESR and low titre rheumatoid factor (RF) positivity may be nonspecific findings in the elderly. Age, gender, duration of disease and symmetric polyarthritis were predictive of poor outcomes in RA. Other poor predictive factors were seropositivity, cervical sublaxation, poor grip strength and early erosive changes.

Treatment

As in OA, nonpharmacological treatment plays an important role, specific treatment with disease modifying drugs like low dose methotrexate is as useful as in adults, though greater care in follow-up is needed due to an increase in ADRs. Antimalarials are a safe second line drugs. A combination therapy of 2 or 3 drugs is effective in resistant RA in adults. Corticosteroids in low doses for elderly patients are useful but with ADRs like osteoporosis, infections are more likely. The tolerability and cost benefit profile of newer drugs like Leflunomide and TNF blocking drugs have to be evaluated in the elderly.

Connective Tissue Diseases: Common in elderly are SLE, Polymyalgia Rheumatica (PMR) and Giant cell arthritis.

SLE: The incidence of SLE in the aged is variable. In the west it ranges between 7 and 18 per cent. While in India it is reportedly 7–8 per cent.[69] Female preponderance may wane with advancing age. Interstitial Lung disease, fever, joint manifestations, thrombocytopenia occur early and are common. Involvement of skin, CNS or kidney is less frequent. Anti-double standard DNA and anti-nuclear antibodies (ANA) titre is lower.[70] Evaluation of lupus is difficult in older patients due to nonspecific symptoms such as joint pains with low titre ANA. ACR diagnostic criteria for SLE are useful to differentiate it from chronic infections, PMR. Treatment of SLE is similar to younger adults but more attention has to be paid to ADRs.

Polymyalgia Rheumatica (PMR)

Commonly affects whites of European descent, with female preponderance (3:1 ratio), blacks and Asians are spared. The prevalence of PMR is approximately 20 per 1,00,000 in over the 50 years of age group. Mean age of onset is 70 years and diagnosis is uncommon below 60 years.[58]

Clinical Features

It is characterized by low grade fever, weight loss, malaise and fatigue. There is pain and proximal muscle stiffness in one or more of three areas, neck, shoulder or hip girdle. Stiffness is marked in early morning and shoulder girdle is most common site. Onset is usually insidious but may be acute in some cases. Movement accelerates pain which is severe at night. There may be stiffness and painful restriction of active movements but passive movements are preserved and there is no atrophy. Some patients may have symmetrical small joint arthritis along with classical features of PMR. Affected joints particularly the knee and sternoclavicular joints are actively inflamed. There are no diagnostic tests but ESR is usually very high (>50mm/min), with normocytic normochronic anaemia, and along with clinical features it is diagnostic. In some cases where ESR may be normal, a high CRP is diagnostic. PMR responds to low dose of steroids (Prednisone); the usual dose is 15–20mg/day for 4 weeks, absence of response by 72 hrs and incomplete response up to 7 days should warrant alternate diagnosis (Box 5). The dose is tapered slowly over months and the lowest effective dose is maintained for 1 year or more. Early withdrawal may result in a relapse. Non treatment of PMR with steroid, may result in giant cell arteritis causing blindness.

Box 5 ***Diseases Mimicking PMR***

Cervical spondylosis	Systemic vasculitis
Rheumatoid arthritis	Inflammatory myopathy (Inclusion body myositis)
Hypothyroidism	Malignancy
Fibromyalgia	

Giant Cell Arteritis: is a localized form of PMR, is uncommon and affects 10 per cent with patients of PMR.[57] Its incidence is 1:1000 in people over 60 years, with a predilection for arteries of the head, particularly the external carotid and retinal branches of internal carotid arteries, more commonly in elderly women (F:M – 3:1).[71] There is an early leucocytoclastic vasculitis followed by chronic inflammation with giant cells in vessel wall. Thrombosis is common, followed by fibrosis. There is familial aggregation and association with HLA-DR4.[72]

Clinical Features

The patient may have an abrupt or insidious onset over weeks or months. Headache is usually first symptom, localized to temporal or occipital region with scalp tenderness. Jaw pain, brought on by chewing or talking, may be the presenting symptom due to ischemia of masseters. Vasculitis of post-ciliary artery leads to occlusion and acute ischemic optic neuropathy. Damage to the optic nerve results in loss of visual acuity and field, reduced colour perception and papillary defects. Sudden visual symptoms in one eye leading rapidly to blindness, is the most common pattern. Fundoscopy may be normal in first 24–36 hrs, once blindness has occurred steroids have no role except preventing blindness in another eye. Sometimes there may be TIAs, brain stem infarcts or hemiparesis. Constitutional symptoms of fatigue, malaise, fever, weight loss, anorexia may be associated. The external carotid artery is characteristically pulseless, firm and tortuous. Arterial biopsy may show typical histological appearance, because of the local nature of the disease and the nonspecific features, the diagnostic yield is low,[73] and there is poor correlation between biopsy findings and disease activity,[73] hence, biopsy is not recommended. Arteriograms may be abnormal but are not done usually. ESR is markedly elevated as in PMR. In some cases ESR may be normal, especially in acute presentations but the CRP may be elevated, which is helpful in diagnosis. There is a good response to high dose steroid therapy (60mg/day). Hence, clinical features, elevated ESR and good response to steroid forms troika for diagnosis. Early management is important to prevent optic artery thrombosis and blindness. After 4–6 weeks of therapy the steroid dosages are tapered to 10–15 mg per day and further tapered by 1 mg per month, in case of recurrence of headache or visual disturbance, a high dose steroid is reinstituted. A maintenance dose is required for a minimum of 1 yr or in some cases life long. Relapse occurs in almost 30 per cent patients and frequent relapses are an indication for corticosteroid sparing agents, which shall be considered if maintenance dose is high (more than 7.5 mg) or with unacceptable ADRs.

Notes

1. R. Yung. "Musculoskeletal disease in the elderly", in D.E. Rosenblatt and V.S. Natarajan (eds.), *Primer on Geriatric Care*. Pixel Studio, Cochin, 2002; 190–208.
2. M. Abrams. *Three Score Years and Ten*. Age Concern, London, 1977.
3. E. Bagge, A. Bjelle, S. Eden and A. Svanborg. "A longitudinal study of the occurrence of joint complaints in elderly people". *Age Ageing*, 1992; 21: 160–167.
4. M.L. Jenkinson, M.R. Bliss, A.T. Brain and D.L. Scott. "Peripheral arthritis in the elderly: A hospital study". *Ann Rheum Dis*, 1989; 48: 227–231.
5. C.P. Schwab. "Arthritis and musculoskeletal pain in elderly", in M.A. Forciea and R.J. Lavizzo-Mourey (eds.), *Geriatric Secrets*. Jaypee Brothers, New Delhi, 1996; 38–44.
6. K.P. Shukla, C.P. Mishra and G. Shanker. "Distribution and role impairment of elderly population in rural area of Varanasi", in D.S. Singh, I.S. Gambhir and A.K. Singh (eds.), *Trends in Geriatric Medicine*. Tara Printing Works, Varanasi, 1996; 284–291.
7. D.L. Scott. "Arthritis in elderly", in R.C. Tallis, H.M. Fillit and J.C. Brocklehurst (eds.), *Brocklehurst's Textbook of Geriatric Medicine and Gerontology*. (5th Ed.), Churchill Livingstone, London, pp. 1155–1178.
8. R.M. Acheson and A.B. Collart. "New Haven survey of joint diseases. XVII: Relationship between some systemic characteristics and osteoarthritis in a general population". *Ann Rheum Dis*, 1975; 34: 379–387.
9. J.L.C.M. Van Saase, L.K.J. Van Romunde, A. Cats et al. "Epidemiology of osteoarthritis: Zoetmeer survey, Comparison of radiological osteoarthritis in a Dutch population with that in 10 other populations". *Ann Rheum Dis*, 1989; 48: 271–280.

10. D.T. Felson. "The epidemiology of osteoarthritis: Results from the Framingham Osteoarthritis Study". *Semin Arthritis Rheum*, 1990; 20 (Suppl. 1): 42–50.
11. A.N. Malviya, R.R. Singh et al. "Prevalence of rheumatic diseases in India: Results of a population survey". *J Ind Rheum Assoc*. 1994; 2: 13–17.
12. D.T. Felson, Y. Zhang, M.T. Hannan et al. "The incidence and natural history of knee osteoarthritis in the elderly: The Framingham Osteoarthritis Study". *Arthritis Rheum*, 1995; 38: 1500–1505.
13. P. Bettica, G. Cline, D.J. Hart, J. Meyer and T.D. Spector. "Evidence for increased bone resorption in patients with progressive knee osteoarthritis: Longitudinal results from the Chingford study". *Arthritis Rheum*, 2002; 46: 3178–3184.
14. R.W. Moskowitz. "Osteoarthritis symptoms and signs", in R.W. Moskowitz, V. Goldberg and H.J. Mankin (eds.), *Osteoarthritis Diagnosis and Management*. WB Saunders Co., Philadelphia, 1993; 255–281.
15. K.D. Brandt. "Osteoarthritis", in D.L. Kasper, E. Braunwald, A. Fauci, S.L. Hauser, D.L. Longo and J.L. Jameson (eds.), *Harrison's Principles of Internal Medicine*. McGraw-Hill, Medical Publishing Division, New York, (16th Ed.), 2005; 2036–2045.
16. D.T. Felson. "The epidemiology of knee osteoarthritis: Result from the Framingham osteoarthritis study". *Semin Arthritis and Rheum*, 1990; 20(Suppl. 3): 42–50.
17. J. Rebort and T.A. Burch. Prevalence of osteoarthritis in adults by age, sex, race and geographic area. United States 1960–62. National Center for Health Statistics, Data from the National Health Survey. Washington DC, United States Government Printing Office, 1996; United States Public Health Service Publication No. 1000, Series 11, No. 15.
18. F.M. Cicuttini and T.D. Spector. "Genetics of osteoarthritis". *Ann Rheum Dis*, 1996; 55: 665–7.
19. A.M. Lievense, S.M.A. Bierma-Zeinstra, A.P. Verhagen, M.E. Van Baar1, J.A.N. Verhaar2 and B.W. Koes. "Influence of obesity on the development osteoarthritis of the hip: A systematic review". *Rheumatology*, 2002; 41: 1155–1162.
20. D.T. Felson. "The course of osteoarthritis and the factors that affect it". *Rheum Dis Clin Nor Am*, 1993; 19: 607–15.
21. N.E. Lane and J.A. Buckwalter. "Exercise: A cause of osteoarthritis?" *Rheum Dis Clin Nor Am*, 1993; 19: 617–32.
22. P. Croft, D. Coggan, M. Cruddas, et al. "Osteoarthritis of the hip: An occupational disease in farmers". *Br Med Journal*, 1992; 304: 1269–72.
23. M. Dougados, A. Gueguen, M. Nguyen, et al. "Longitudinal radiologic evaluation of osteoarthritis of the knee". *J Rheum*, 1992; 19: 378–83.

24. V.B. Kraus. "Pathogenesis and treatment of osteoarthritis". *Med Clin Nor Am*, 1997; 81: 85–112.
25. J. Cushnahan and P.A. Dieppe. "Study of 500 patients with limb joint osteoarthritis. I. Analysis by age, sex and distribution of symptomatic joint sites". *Ann Rheum Dis*, 1991; 50: 8–13.
26. Z.S. Rosenberg, S. Shankman, G.C. Steiner et al. "Rapid destructive osteoarthritis: Clinical, radiographic, and pathologic features". *Radiology*, 1992; 182: 213–216.
27. K.D. Brandt. "A pessimistic view of serologic markers for diagnosis and management of osteoarthirits. Biochemical immunologics and clinicopathologic barriers". *J Rheumatol*, 1989; 18: 39–42.
28. R. Altman, E. Asch, D. Bloch et al. "Development of criteria for the classification and reporting of osteoarthritis". *Arthritis Rheum*, 1986; 29: 1039–49.
29. R. Altman, G. Alarcon, D. Applerouth et al. "The American College of Rheumatology: Criteria for the classification and reporting of hip". *Arthritis Rheumatism*, 1991; 34: 505–14.
30. R. Altman, G. Alarcon, D. Applerouth et al. "The American College of Rheumatology: Criteria for the classification and reporting of hand". *Arthritis Rheum*, 1990; 33: 1601–10.
31. T. McAlindon and P. Dieppe. "Osteoarthritis definitions and criteria". *Ann Rheum Dis*, 1989; 48: 531–532.
32. M.D. Hochberg, R. Altman, K.D. Brandt et al. "Guidelines for the medical management of osteoarthritis – Part I. Osteoarthritis of the hip". *Arthritis Rheum*, 1995; 38: 1535–40.
33. M.D. Hochberg, R. Altman, K.D. Brandt et al. "Guidelines for the medical management of osteoarthritis – Part II. Osteoarthritis of the knee". *Arthritis Rheum*, 1995; 38: 1541–6.
34. N. Watts. "Changes in BMD and RR for fracture". *J Bone Minor Res*, 1999; 14 (Suppl. 1): S136.
35. P. Dieppe, J. Chard and P. Juri. "The management of osteoarthritis". *NEJM*, (in press).
36. F. Wolfe, S. Zhao and N. Lane. "Preference fornonsteroidal anti-inflammatory drugs over acetaminophen by rheumatic disease patients: survey of 1,799 patients with osteoarthritis, rheumatoid arthritis, and fibromyalgia". *Arthritis Rheum*, 2000; 43: 378–85.
37. T. Pincus, G.G. Koch, T. Sokka, J. Lefkowith, F. Wolfe, J.M. Jordan et al. "A randomized, double-blind, crossover clinical trial of diclofenac plus misoprostol versus acetaminophen in patients with osteoarthritis of the hip or knee". *Arthritis Rheum*, 2001; 44: 1587–98.

38. D.J. Levinson and H.M. Rubinstein. "Double blind comparison of fenoprofen calcium and ibuprofen in osteoarthritis of large joints". *Curr Ther Res*, 1983; 34: 280–4.
39. B.J. Lister, M. Poland and R.E. DeLapp. "Efficacy of nabumetone versus diclofenac, naproxen, ibuprofen, and piroxicam in osteoarthritis and rheumatoid arthritis". *Am J Med*, 1993; 95: 2–9S.
40. L.S. Simon, F.L. Lanza, P.E. Lipsky, R.C. Hubbard, S. Talwalker, B.D. Schwartz et al. "Preliminary study of the safety and efficacy of SC-58365, a novel cyclooxygenase 2 inhibitor". *Arthritis Rheum*, 1998; 41: 1591–602.
41. K. Saag, C. Fisher, J. McKay et al. "For the MK-0966 Phase III Protocol 033 Study Group. MK-0966, a specific Cox-2 inhibitor, has clinical efficacy comparable to ibuprofen in the treatment of knee and hip osteoarthritis in a 6-week controlled clinical trial". *Arthritis Rheum*, 1998; 41 (Suppl. 9): S196.
42. G.P. Geba, A.L. Weaver, A.B. Polis, M.E. Dixon and T.J. Schnitzer. "Efficacy of rofecoxib, celecoxib, and acetaminophen in osteoarthritis of the knee". *JAMA*, 2002; 287: 64–71.
43. F.E. Silverstein, G. Faich, J.L. Goldstein, L.S. Simon, T. Pincus, A. Whelton et al. "Gastrointestinal toxicity with celecoxib vs nonsteroidal antiinflammatorydrugs for osteoarthritis and rheumatoid arthritis. The CLASS Study: A randomized controlled trial". *JAMA*, 2000; 284: 1247–55.
44. F. Silverstein, D.Y. Graham, J.R. Senior, H.W. Davies, B.J. Struthers, R.M. Bittman et al. "Misoprostol reduces serious gastrointestinal complications in patients with rheumatoid arthritis receiving nonsteroidal anti-inflammatory drugs: A randomized, double-blind, placebo-controlled trial". *Ann Intern Med*, 1995; 123: 241–9.
45. G. Singh and D.R. Ramey. "NSAID inducedgastrointestinal complications: The ARAMIS perspective – 1997". *J Rheumatol*, 1998; 25 (Suppl.): 8–16.
46. W.B. Katz. "Progress with tramadol: US experience". *Clin Courier,* 1997; 14: 1–12.
47. T. McAlindon. "An evaluation of glucosamine for the treatment of OA", in K.D. Brandt, M.A. Doherty, R.B. Raffa, M.R. Griffin, M.A. Minor, M. Liang et al. "Proceedings of Symposium: Controversies and Practical Issues in the Management of Osteoarthritis. Part 3". *J Clin Rheumatol,* (in press).
48. K.D. Brandt, S.A. Mazzuca, B.P. Katz and K.A. Lane. "Doxycycline Study Group: The disease modifying effect of doxycycline (doxy) includes symptomatic benefit for patients with knee osteoarthritis". *Arthritis Rheum*, 2003; 48: 3643.
49. T.D. Spector, P.G. Conaghan, J.C. Buckland-Wright et al. "Effect of risedronate on joints structure and symptoms of knee osteoarthritis: Results of the BRISK randomized, controlled trial". *Arthritis Research and Therapy*, 2005; 7: R625–R633.

50. C. Bingham, J. Beary, S. Cohen, D. Clauw, G. Cline and J. Meyer. "Clinically significant placebo improvement occurs by 6 months and is maintained through 24 months in a study of knee OA pain and function". American College of Rheumatology, Annual Meeting, October 16–21, 2004; San Antonio, TX 2004; 263.
51. K. Pavelka, J. Gatterova, M. Olejarova, S. Machacek, G. Giacovelli and L.C. Rovati. "Glucosamine sulfate use and delay of progression of knee osteoarthritis". *Arch Intern Med*, 2002; 162: 2113–23.
52. S.A. Mazzuca, K.D. Brandt, K.A. Lane and B.P. Katz. "Knee pain reduces joint space width in conventional standing anteroposterior radiographs of osteoarthritic knees". *Arthritis Rheum*, 2002; 46: 1223–7.
53. J.C. Buckland-Wright, F. Wolfe, R.J. Ward, N. Flowers and C. Hayne. "Substantial superiority of semiflexed (MTP) views in knee osteoarthritis: A comparative radiographic study, without fluoroscopy, of standing extended, semiflexed AP, and schuss views". *J Rheumatol*, 1999; 26: 2664–74.
54. S.A. Mazzuca, K.D. Brandt and K.A. Buckwalter. "Detection of radiographic joint space narrowing in subjects with knee osteoarthritis: Longitudinal comparison of the metatarsophalangeal and semiflexed anteroposterior view". *Arthritis Rheum*, 2003; 48: 385–90.
55. D.A. Freund and R.S. Dittus. Assessing and improving outcomes: Total knee replacement. Final report of the patient outcomes research team (PORT), Washington: AHCPR Pub., No 97-N015, 1997.
56. I. Wiklund and B. Romanus. "A comparison of quality of life before and after arthroplasty in patients who had arthrosis of the hip joint". *J Bone Joint Surg Am*, 1991; 73: 765–9.
57. M. Doherty, P. Lanyon and R.H. Ralston. "Musculoskeletal disorders", in C. Harlett, E.R. Chilvers, N.A. Boon and N.R. Colledge (eds.), *Davidson's Principles and Practice of Medicine*. Churchill Livingstone, Edinburg, London, New York, (19th Ed.), 2002, pp. 1017–1019 (CPPD), 1015–1016 (Gout), 1040–1042 (PMR).
58. D.T. Felson, J.J. Anderson, A. Naimarka, W. Cannel and R.F. Meenan. "The prevalence of chondrocalcinosis in the elderly and its association with knee osteoarthritis: The Framingham Study". *J Rheumatol*, 1989; 16: 1241–1245.
59. R.A. Mayer, D.C. Bush and T.M. Harrington. "Acute calcific tendonitis of the hand and writs". *J Rheumatol*, 1989; 16: 198–202.
60. R.S. Pinals and C.L. Short. "Calcific periarthritis involving multiple sites". *Arthritis Rheum*, 1966; 9: 566–574.
61. D.J. MeCarty, P.B. Halverson, G.F. Carrera et al. "Milwakee shoulder association of microsteroids containing hydroxyapactite crystals, active collagenase and neutral protease with rotator cuff defects". *Arthritis Rheum*, 1981; 24: 464–491.

62. G.V. Campion, F. MeCrae, W. Alwan et al. "Idiopathic destructive arthritis of the shoulder". *Semin Arthritis Rheum*, 1988; 70: 232–245.
63. A. Engel, J. Roberts and T.A. Burch. "Rheumatoid arthritis in adults: United States, 1960–1962". *Vital and Health Statistics*, National Centre for Health Statistics, DHEW, Series 11, No. 17, 1966.
64. L.A. Healey. "Rheumatoid arthritis in elderly". *Clin Rheum Dis.*, 1986; 12: 173–179.
65. A.N. Chandrasekaran, B. Radhakrishna et al. "Spectrum of clinical and immunological features of systemic rheumatic disorders in a referral hospital in South India-Rheumatoid arthritis". *J Ind Rheum Assoc.*, 1994; 2: 18–26.
66. H.R. Schumacher. "Palindromic onset of rheumatoid arthritis". *Arthritis Rheum*, 1982; 25: 361–369.
67. A.B. Hassell, M.J. Davis and P.D. Fowler. "The relationship between serial measures of disease activity and outcome in rheumatoid arthritis". *QJ Med.*, 1993; 86: 601–607.
68. H.S. Meena, A. Kumar and R. Muralidhar. "Spectrum of inflammatory joint disease in elderly and clinical profile of late onset rheumatoid arthritis". *J Ind Rheum Ass.*, 1995; 3: 4–7.
69. A. Wilson, M.E. Hamilton, D.A. Spyker et al. "Age influences the clinical and serological expression of SLE". *Arthr Rheum*, 1981; 24: 1230–1235.
70. A.J. Fremont. "Connective Tissue Disease", in R.C. Tallis, H.M. Fillit and J.C. Brocklehurst (eds.), *Brocklehurst's Textbook of Geriatric Medicine and Gerontology*. (5th Ed.), Churchill Livingstone, London, pp. 1179–1187.
71. J.D. Bignon, J. Barrier, J.P. Soulillou et al. "HLA DR4 and giant cell arteritis". *Tissue Antigens*, 1984; 24: 60–62.
72. N.C. Mambo. "Temporal (granulomatous) arteritis: A histopathological study of 32 cases". *Histopathology*, 1970; 3: 209–221.
73. K.A. Huston, G.G. Hunder, J.T. Lie et al. "Temporal arteritis: A 25-year epidemoilogic, clinical and pathologic study". *Ann Intern Med*, 1978; 88: 162–167.

6 Dementia and Alzheimer's Disease

M.K. Thakur

Dementia is one of the greatest public health and social challenges. It is a neurological disorder that affects the ability to think, speak, reason, remember and move. It is a progressive brain dysfunction, which results in a restriction of daily activities and in most cases leads to the need for long-term care. It affects not only patients, but also those related to them and on whom the patients depend for care. There are three most common forms of dementia – Alzheimer's disease (AD), vascular dementia and Lewy body dementia. Sometimes, a person can have more than one of these problems at the same time. Some of these disorders get worse with time and cannot be cured, whereas other types can be treated and reversed.

In vascular dementia, arteries feeding the brain become narrowed or blocked. The onset of symptoms is usually abrupt, frequently occurring after a stroke. Some forms of vascular dementia progress slowly, making them difficult to distinguish from AD. Some people have Alzheimer's and vascular dementia simultaneously. Vascular dementia often causes problems with thinking, language, walking, bladder control and vision. The progression of vascular dementia may be halted after preventing additional strokes by treating the underlying diseases such as high blood pressure. In Lewy body dementia, abnormal round structures called Lewy bodies develop within cells of the midbrain, beneath the cerebral hemispheres. It shares characteristics with both AD and Parkinson's disease. Like AD, it causes confusion and impaired memory and judgement. It often produces two distinctive physical signs typical of Parkinson's disease – a shuffling gait and flexed posture.

Lewy body dementia can also cause hallucinations. Lewy bodies contain a protein associated with Parkinson's disease, and they are often found in the brains of people who have Parkinson's disease or AD. This suggests that the three ailments are related, or that Lewy body dementia and Alzheimer's or Parkinson's disease sometimes co-exist in the same person. Some people with Lewy body dementia have experienced dramatic improvements in symptoms when treated with medications for Alzheimer's or Parkinson's disease.

The most common and well-known type of dementia is AD, which was first described in 1907 by the German physician Alois Alzheimer. AD is more severe than the mild memory loss that many people experience as they grow older. It is a progressive degenerative disease that affects areas of the brain involved in memory, intelligence, judgement, language and behaviour. It causes memory loss, disorientation, depression and decay of bodily functions. It is characterized by a deterioration of both cognitive and physical abilities. It first affects memory and the ability to carry out complex, coordinated tasks. It also causes depression, inattention and outbursts of anger. It affects personality, the ability to think clearly, and the ability to carry out daily activities. In a more progressive stage, the disease can cause difficulties in the ability to perform even simple tasks such as speaking and comprehending, eating and sleeping. The affected person can even forget his name and identity (Thakur, 2000, 2002).

Prevalence of Alzheimer's Disease

Dementia predominantly occurs in the second half of lifespan, often after the age of 65 years. Probably this is the 'price society has to pay' for higher life expectancy and therefore the term 'dementia' causes fear and repression similar to the terms 'cancer' or 'AIDS'. The probability of suffering from dementia increases with advancing age from less than 2 per cent for the 65–69-year olds, to 5 per cent for the 75–79-year olds and to more than 20 per cent for the 85–89 year olds and about 30 per cent of those over 90. Every third person over 90 years of age suffers from moderate or severe dementia. About half of those affected by dementia suffer from AD. Since the average life span has increased over the years, AD is becoming a more common problem. The probability is higher for women and for people having a lower standard of education. More than 18 million people are affected with dementia worldwide. Out of them, AD afflicts about 12 million people including more than 4 million Americans and over 3 million Indians (Bagchi, 2002). It is increasing so fast that more than 22 million people worldwide will be affected by 2025.

What Causes Alzheimer's Disease?

Many complex diseases develop through interactions among genetic, environmental and lifestyle factors. The importance of these factors may differ from person to person. AD is one of these complex diseases. It develops over many years, and it appears to be affected by a number of factors that may increase or decrease a person's risk of developing the disease. Though we do not have control over some of the risk factors for AD like age and genes, we can take care of other possible risk factors.

The biggest risk for Alzheimer's is simply age. Alzheimer's cases double with every five years of age between 65 and 85. Although most people who develop AD do not have a family history of the condition, one is at increased risk for the condition if a member of the family has it.

In a small percentage of cases, the disease is caused by genetic changes (mutations) in the family. Scientists have found genetic links to the two forms of AD. Early-onset AD is a very rare form of the disease that can occur in people between the age of 30 and 60. In the 1980s and the early 1990s, researchers found that mutations (or changes) in amyloid precursor protein (APP), presenilin (PS)1 and PS2 genes located on three different chromosomes cause early-onset AD. A person has a 50–50 chance of developing early-onset AD if one parent has any of these genetic mutations. Late-onset AD, the more common form, develops after age 65. In 1992, researchers found that certain forms of the apolipoprotein E (apoE) gene can influence AD risk. For example, apoE2, a rarely occurring form, may provide some protection; apoE3, the most common form, appears to play a neutral role; and apoE4, which is found in about 40 per cent of people with AD, appears to increase the risk. However, merely having the apoE4 gene does not mean that a person will definitely develop AD; it only increases the risk. If a patient has dementia, the presence of apoE4 increases the likelihood that the dementia is due to AD. There are also many cases where people develop AD without having an apoE4 gene.

APP is cleaved by proteases to produce a small peptide beta amyloid which can accumulate in the spaces between brain cells and form plaques in the brain. These plaques are associated with the death of brain cells, causing a gradual loss of memory and control of body function, and leading eventually to death. By the time a patient has noticeable symptoms of Alzheimer's, substantial amounts of amyloid have accumulated in the brain and this destroys the nerve cells. The slowly progressing destruction of nerve cells leads to the symptoms of AD. It is a natural phenomenon to lose a certain number of nerve cells during ageing but this loss occurs much more rapidly in people suffering from AD. As a result, the brain of the patient does not function normally any longer. Scientists have discovered a link between a prominent developmental gene and neurovascular dysfunction in AD. The gene plays a major role in the growth and remodelling of vascular systems. However, the expression of this gene is low in brain cells of people with AD. In laboratory studies, scientists showed that restoration of the gene expression level in the human brain cells stimulated the formation of new blood vessels. It also increased the level of a protein that removes amyloid beta peptide. In further studies, scientists deleted one copy of the gene in mice and found that such mice have reduced ability to grow blood vessels in the brain and impaired clearance of amyloid beta. This gene is a homeobox gene known as $MEOX_2$ and also as GAX, which encodes proteins that determine development. The expression of $MEOX_2$ or mesenchyme homeobox 2, is low in human brain endothelial cells taken from autopsy samples of Alzheimer patients. When the expression of $MEOX_2$ is low, apoptosis or programmed cell death occurs in the brain's vascular system.

In recent years, it has been shown that another pathological process that occurs in the brain of AD patients is excessive immune activation and inflammation, which is induced by overproduction of an inflammation-producing protein called interleukin-1, as well as a few other related compounds. This process can impair the functioning of nerve cells and even lead to their death. Furthermore, genetic alterations in the interleukin-1 gene have been associated with increased risk for the appearance and severity of AD symptoms. Some population studies suggest an association between a reduced risk of AD and NSAIDs, such as ibuprofen, naproxen and indomethacin (Cole et al., 2004). Over the last few years, association of Alzheimer's with lifestyle has emerged. Scientists have found that what is good for the heart may also be good for the brain. The risk factors for heart disease—high blood pressure, diabetes, excess weight, high cholesterol and lack of exercise—may also play a role in AD. In recent years, basic research in laboratories as well as population and animal studies have suggested a close connection between AD risk and high levels of cholesterol and high blood pressure (Kivipelto et al., 2002; Sjogren and Blennow, 2005). High cholesterol can narrow the arteries and raise the risk of heart disease. Similarly high cholesterol may also affect brain arteries and promote clumping of the beta-amyloid peptide, which causes neurodegeneration in Alzheimer's. A recent population study has shown that people who take statins, the most commonly prescribed cholesterol lowering drugs, have reduced risk of developing dementia (Kivipelto et al., 2005). Moderately elevated levels of insulin increase the concentration of inflammatory markers and beta amyloid in plasma and cerebrospinal fluid, and these markers may contribute to AD. Mark A. Fishel and colleagues (2005) raised blood insulin levels (while maintaining normal blood sugar levels) in 16 healthy older adults ranging in age from 55 to 81 years, and then measured the changes in levels of inflammatory markers, modulators and beta-amyloid in plasma and cerebrospinal fluid. Moderate peripheral hyperinsulinemia (increased levels of insulin) provoked striking increases in CNS (central nervous system) inflammatory markers. Thus, the findings suggest that insulin-resistant conditions such as diabetes mellitus and hypertension may increase the risk for AD, in part through insulin-induced inflammation. Another finding has shown that a high level of the amino acid homocysteine is associated with an increased risk of developing AD. High levels of homocysteine are known to increase heart disease risk, and make neurons stop working and die (Irizarry et al., 2005, Ravaglia et al., 2005).

Symptoms of Alzheimer's Disease

The most commonly known symptom of AD is confusion. People suffering from this disease usually forget, misplace, cannot remember names, cannot find their own cars in the car park and/or experience similar lapses. They suffer mainly from impaired memory and orientation, limitations of concentration, planning and judgement, personality changes, and later they also suffer perceptual, speech and walking disorders. In the final stage, various other body functions such as swallowing and the excretion process are also affected. Close family members usually notice symptoms first, although the person affected also may realize that something is wrong. As the disease progresses, the symptoms get worse. The person may also develop strange new behaviours and withdraw from family and friends. Hallucinations, delusions and paranoia are common; some people may become verbally or physically aggressive or abusive. Eventually, the person may forget how to perform basic tasks such as eating, dressing, bathing, using the toilet, or getting up from a bed or chair and walking. The patients gradually lose their independence in managing everyday life. There are effects on perception and social relationships; people become more and more dependent on care. The most important early indications of dementia include:

1. *Forgetfulness (anomia):* Most people sometimes forget names or appointments. If this happens more frequently and inexplicable states of confusion also occur, this might be an indication of a decline in memory function.
2. *Language problems (aphasia):* Most people sometimes experience difficulties in finding the right words. Dementia sufferers often cannot remember simple words and instead they use inappropriate fillers which make it difficult to understand their sentences.
3. *Problems with spatial and temporal orientation (agnosia):* Several people sometimes forget the day of the week or they get lost in unfamiliar surroundings. Dementia sufferers might be in their own street and no longer know where they are, how they got there and how to get home again.
4. *Impaired capacity of judgement (apraxia):* Dementia sufferers sometimes wear totally inappropriate clothes. For example, they wear a bathrobe while shopping or several blouses on top of each other on a hot summer day.
5. *Problem with abstract thinking:* For many people, running a bank account is a challenge. Dementia patients can often neither recognise numbers nor carry out simple calculations.
6. *Mood swings and behavioural changes:* Everybody has mood swings. People with dementia may have very sudden mood swings, often without discernible cause.
7. *Personality changes:* With advancing age, the personality of most people changes a little. People affected by dementia may experience a very pronounced personality change suddenly or over a longer period of time. Somebody who is generally friendly, for example, becomes unexpectedly angry, jealous or timid.
8. *Loss of initiative:* Nobody continuously works with the same motivation. Dementia patients sometimes lose their zest for work and their interest in hobbies completely without enjoying new activities.

Stages of Alzheimer's Disease

Alzheimer's disease is a slowly unfolding, progressive disease which is accompanied over time by changes in the appearance of the patient. As this progression tends to be accompanied by distinct symptoms, the disease is typically divided into three stages: (1) mild or early stage, characterized by impaired mental ability as well as mood swings, (2) moderate or mid-stage when behavioural disturbances develop, and (3) advanced or late stage, physical problems are dominant.

The Early Stage

During this stage, the patient and carer are confronted with a number of symptoms that can be very distressing for both patient and carer as they struggle to understand the symptoms and diagnosis of the disease.

Memory and intellectual capacity seem to become increasingly affected. The patient forgets more and more and the most recent events seem to be forgotten most quickly.

Language and perception deteriorate as patients can't find the right words and can't understand the conversation or interpret the events they are witnessing. So the patients start to resort to shouting and touching as means of communication.

Functioning and dealing with daily life actions such as using a spoon or getting dressed become more and more difficult. The inability to think in an abstract way coupled with impaired judgement mean that connecting thoughts are no longer understood or recognized.

Perception and feelings: AD patients lose skills and abilities as well as the capacity to interact, suggesting a change in personality. Dementia doesn't change a person, but is a process that brings changes in the existence of the person involved. Sometimes characteristics that had been buried can surface. For example, a person who was always very gentle suddenly shows aggressive behaviour. People with dementia lose their perception of time. The patients live and experience their environment in an inextricable mixture of inside and outside, past and present, dream and reality. Patients live in their own 'other' world of scenes, people and situations.

The more the disease progresses, the more the people become dependent on their environment and the people they directly relate to. One of the most distressing things for the carer is to witness their relative losing control and being more and more at the mercy of his/her own body and feelings.

The Mid Stage

A stage of confusion: People with dementia slowly move from forgetfulness into confusion and therefore also into a new, different, initially strange and threatening mode of being. The person lives more and more in his/her *own, dreamlike 'world'* in which present and past blend together and in which the rules and structures of the 'old world' – what is right, what is important – lose importance. At this stage people with dementia increasingly see themselves not as confused in a logical environment, but as oriented in a very unfamiliar and confusing environment.

Communication: The increasing loss of memory leads a patient to understanding less and less of what others say to him/her. Vocabulary becomes limited and verbal communication is characterized by mixed-up words, swapping of syllables and short sentences. People with dementia increasingly resort to physical, non-verbal communication.

Aggressive behaviour of the patient: Trivial events or small failures can cause a sudden change in mood which can result in screaming, scolding and/or kicking. The patient generally reacts to fears, excessive demands, frustrations and misunderstandings. This aggression often disappears after a few minutes and the patient gets very confused if the aggressive behaviour is mentioned. Darkness, odours, high room temperature and noisy confusing sounds, boredom or overstimulation (blaring radio, running television) favour aggressive outbursts. This in turn can frighten relatives of Alzheimer patients as people with dementia often retain their physical strength.

The Late Stage

Helplessness: In the third stage of the disease, also called severe AD, patients become more and more helpless and dependent. Access to their 'bubble'-like world in which they hide and retreat becomes more difficult as language deteriorates. Their memory has gone and *repetitive movements* might emerge such as rocking, undressing, and walking up and down. Often people become increasingly *rigid* towards the end of their life and their face becomes expressionless and rigid, the jaws are clenched and the body stiffens. This can lead to difficulties with eating and falling.

Confinement to bed: At this stage, the patient is likely to suffer from urine and bowel incontinence. Confinement in bed is linked to many difficulties. Movement has to be encouraged to avoid bedsores and ulcers, immune system deteriorates and infections occur more easily and as people curl up in bed, they develop ankyliosis (or immobility and consolidation of the joints). Clenching of the jaws now becomes a very stressful problem because it is difficult to feed them. The patients increasingly suffer from dysphagia (problems in swallowing), constantly swallows the wrong way and thereby contract pneumonia (aspiration pneumonia).

Diagnosis of Alzheimer's Disease

Alzheimer's disease is diagnosed after a careful medical history and physical examination, evaluation of the person's mental and functional status, and selected laboratory tests and imaging tests, such as CT and MRI scans, to rule out other possible causes of the symptoms. Imaging tests may identify subtle changes in the structures of the brain that may relate to AD, but they may not provide enough evidence for a diagnosis (Lee et al., 2003). Part of the first examination includes laboratory blood tests and possibly cerebral liquor tests. There is an urgent need for simple, specific tests that will enable the average family doctor to reliably identify the disease, especially in the early or even pre-symptomatic stages when medicines might be most effective. Some physicians also carry out electroencephalography (EEG) or imaging diagnostics such as computer or nuclear spin tomography (magnetic resonance tomography, MRT) which show the brain in layers or even in its function (for example positron emission tomography, PET). These studies show that MRI and PET scans or other imaging or biological markers can be used to identify early AD changes and disease progression. These tests may help to identify those people who are at risk of AD before they develop symptoms as well as help physicians assess the response to treatment. Patients affected by dementia are usually not able to visit a physician on their own initiative. This is where the support of the relatives is important. The physician will conduct a general physical and neurological examination in addition to documenting the medical history. In addition, a series of examination procedures are conducted involving psychometric tests, sometimes with questionnaires or a few exercises. This serves to establish the extent of the difficulties. Part of such a neuropsychological examination includes the Mini-Mental State Examination (MMSE) which is a commonly used test. This procedure can be a strain for the patient. During such examinations, the problems become obvious and this can trigger shame and also despair (especially if the relatives are present and the problems have not previously been discussed).

The most important sources of information are those people to whom the patient relates. The physician consults with them concerning the medical history of the patient, similar diseases of relatives, development of current symptoms, limitations in dealing with everyday life and about possible behavioural disturbances or dangers.

Can Dementia be Treated?

As with numerous other diseases, there is no cure for AD but medication can improve disease symptoms. A number of drugs, designed to improve brain function, are available on the market. Typically antidementia or psychotropic drugs are prescribed. Psychotropic drugs can be used as a supportive therapy in the treatment of behavioural problems in dementia. There is often the criticism that these agents are only used to quiet patients down so that they will behave in an apathetic manner, with the result that they cannot take part in daily events. The available drugs are effective but they also influence patients in a negative fashion because of other side effects. An increasing degree of confusion can be caused by physical illness, and restlessness and aggressive behaviour can be connected to pain. Therefore, it is important to observe the general state of health of the patient and treat any underlying conditions. Improving the patient's general condition will improve their feelings of well-being and thereby mitigate their feelings of restlessness and aggression. Recently, substantial progress has been made in the therapy of disturbed dementia patients. Physicians can now treat these patients effectively so that patients are not dozing during the day and wandering around at night.

The medicines administered today to Alzheimer's patients focus on preventing the breakdown of acetylcholine, a chemical produced by brain cells which transmits information within the brain and is vitally involved in cognitive processes that include memory, attention and thought. Because acetylcholine-producing cells are among the first to die in Alzheimer's patients, drug-induced elevation of acetylcholine levels partially attenuates the cognitive deterioration. The more recent antidementia agents belong to the so-called acetylcholinesterase inhibitors such as reminyl (galantamine), exelon (rivastigmine) and aricept (donepezil)). With these drugs the deterioration of the symptoms can be delayed. The Hebrew University researchers found that anti-AD drugs not only block the activity of the enzyme responsible for breaking down acetylcholine but also cause a marked reduction in the production of interleukin-1 (Reale et al., 2005). Furthermore, they describe the use of a novel drug (EN101), which produces these effects in a more efficient way by destroying the messenger RNA of the enzyme, rather than simply blocking the enzyme activity.

Antibody therapy: In recent years, there has been a lot of interest in using antibodies against the abnormal deposits of beta amyloid in the brain. In a study (Oddo et al., 2004), mice were genetically engineered to develop plaques and tangles, and then treated with beta amyloid antibodies. Three days after injection, the immune system of the mice cleared the amyloid and two days later the tangles also disappeared. However, with vaccine research, scientists have at times run into unforeseen problems. A clinical trial of a vaccine based on antibodies was halted in 2002, after some of the people participating in the trial developed encephalitis—a dangerous inflammation of the brain.

Weiner and his colleagues took a different approach, designing a vaccine—administered via drops in the nose—that would initiate an amyloid-cleansing process by triggering the immune system without provoking antibody development. The researchers targeted a specific type of amyloid-eating cells known as microglial cells—stimulating the cells into action to essentially gobble up the amyloid build-up (Shie et al., 2005). Before the study, the mice had a build-up of beta-amyloid plaque in their brains in amounts similar to what would be present in an Alzheimer's patient. The vaccine was administered to the mice on a weekly basis for six weeks, after an initial grouping of four doses was given within the first week. The research team began monitoring the mice one week after vaccination started, looking for signs of disease, paralysis, limb weakness and fatigue. Ultimately, the brain was dissected and examined for evidence of both amyloid quantity and any toxic side effects that might have developed in reaction to the vaccine. The amyloid plaque levels in the vaccinated mice were reduced by 73 per cent and none of the vaccinated mice showed any evidence of encephalitis or other toxic side effects. Although it has so far only been tested on mice, Weiner and his team hoped to begin small-scale testing of the Alzheimer's nasal spray vaccine in people by 2006.

How is Dementia Managed?

Though there is no known cure for AD, a number of studies have indicated that certain substances can slow the progression of the disorder and improve functioning. Obviously, the earlier the intervention, the better is the chance for improvement. Efforts can be made to maintain the quality of life and help the person stay active. With support, education and planning, caregivers may find ways of making life easier for the person they take care of and for themselves.

Treatment focuses on several areas including improving memory and daily functioning, dealing with new and unusual behaviours, and treating other conditions that commonly occur with AD such as depression. Medications, including cholinesterase inhibitors or memantine, may temporarily improve memory and thinking problems.

Other treatment includes making sure the home is safe and providing supportive care as the condition worsens. Managing this disorder or any dementia involves multiple supplemental agents, though there is no "magic pill". Many of the supplements listed here prevent or stop some symptoms of the disease.

Antioxidants prevent and slow dementia: There is overwhelming clinical evidence that antioxidants, which fight against free radicals, are effective in preventing the symptoms of both dementia and Alzheimer's. A recent report suggests that vitamin C and vitamin E supplements may reduce the risk of dementia. Nearly 3,400 Japanese-American men participated in a long-term study. It was found that men who took both vitamins C and E had 88 per cent lower risk of vascular dementia than those who took neither supplement. Bruce Ames and his colleagues at the University of California discovered that acetyl-L-carnitine (ALC) combined with a second antioxidant alpha lipoic acid gave new life to old brain cells (Bianchetti et al., 2003; Ono et al., 2004) have found that vitamin A exhibits potent antiamyloidogenic and fibril-destabilizing effects in vitro.

Some studies have found a correlation between low vitamin B_{12} levels and the development of AD and dementia (Tucker et al., 2005) others have found no such correlation. Researchers from Karolinska Institute provide convincing evidence that a deficiency of either vitamin B_{12} or folic acid (folate) is associated with an increased risk of AD and dementia. Their study involved 370 non-demented people aged 75 years and older who were not supplementing with vitamin B_{12} or folate. The participants were tested at baseline to determine mental status and had blood samples drawn for analysis of vitamin B_{12} and folate levels. Only subjects who showed no signs of dementia were included in the follow-up group. Three years later 77 of the participants had developed dementia; of these 59 were diagnosed with AD. Compared with participants with normal levels of vitamin B_{12} and folate, the participants with low levels of at least one of the vitamins had 2.3 times higher risk of AD and 1.7 times risk of any kind of dementia. These risk estimates were obtained after adjusting for other risk factors such as age, sex and educational attainment. The researchers speculate that vitamin B_{12} and folic acid help prevent this effect by reducing the body levels of homocysteine, a known neurotoxin involved in the development of AD.

Melatonin is miraculous and has many proven benefits. Now its deficiency has been shown to have a strong link to Alzheimer's. A study found that elderly people, who eat fish or seafood even once a week, are at lower risk of developing dementia, including AD. Boosting levels of fatty acid docosahexaenoic acid (DHA) in the blood and eating about three fish meals each week can almost halve the risk of AD in elderly men and women, confirming previous results showing the benefit of fish oils on mental health. Researchers at Tufts University in Boston measured the fatty acid levels in blood samples obtained from 1137 men and women, with an average age of 75. Participants who had diets rich in DHA, an omega-3 fatty acid, reduced their risk of developing dementia considerably compared with those whose diets contained low amounts of DHA.

New research shows that *curcumin*, an extract of the turmeric roots from which Indian curry is derived, may explain why the rates of AD among Indian elderly are 90 per cent lower than in US and Canada (Cole et al., 2001). In rats, curcumin not only reduces the amyloid but also reduces the brain's response to the amyloid. So curcumin is a powerful antioxidant and anti-inflammatory agent. In her study, Frautschy fed adult (9 months) and old (22 months) rats diets rich in curcumin. All the rats had received brain injections of amyloid to mimic progressive AD. Curcumin reduced the accumulation of beta-amyloid and the associated loss of proteins in the synapses or gaps between individual brain cells (Lim et al., 2001). Synapses connect nerve cells and are crucial for memory. Rats fed curcumin performed much better in memory-dependent maze tests compared with rats on normal diets. Curcumin is several times more potent a free radical scavenger than vitamin E (alpha-tocopherol). (Ono et al., 2004) found that curcumin decreases the "fiber-forming ability" of amyloid beta and even dissolves already-fibrous amyloid beta.

A number of population-based studies suggest that lifestyle interventions may help to slow the onset and progression of AD. Scientists are seeking to find out if and how physically or cognitively stimulating activity might delay the onset and progression of AD. As research suggests that high cholesterol may contribute to stroke and brain cell damage, a low fat, low cholesterol diet is advisable. There is growing evidence that a diet rich in dark vegetables and fruits, which contain antioxidants, may help protect brain cells. Social activity not only makes physical and mental activity more enjoyable, it can reduce stress levels, which helps maintain healthy connections among brain cells. Mentally stimulating activities strengthen brain cells and the connections between them, and may even create new nerve cells.

Physical exercise is essential for maintaining good blood flow to the brain as well as to encourage new brain cells so that it responds better to a task or that it activates cellular mechanisms that improve brain function. It can also significantly reduce the risk of heart attack, stroke and diabetes, and thereby protect against those risk factors for Alzheimer's and other dementias (Rovio et al., 2005). In a recent study, Adlard et al (2005) have shown in an animal model system that one simple behavioural interventione – exercise – could delay, or even prevent, development of AD-like pathology by decreasing beta-amyloid levels. Another study found that beta-amyloid levels decreased in the brains of transgenic mice when they were housed in groups and in environments that were enriched with running wheels, coloured tunnels, and toys (Lazarov et al., 2005). Both of these studies are exciting because they offer insight into one of the pathways through which exercise and environment might promote resistance to development of cognitive changes that come with ageing and AD.

Concluding Remarks

Though we can not do much about our age or genetic profile, recent research demonstrates the importance of healthy diet for long-term brain health and suggests that maintaining good health habits may lower the chances of developing several serious diseases including AD. Scientists are studying a number of health, lifestyle and environmental factors that could make a difference. Many of these potential factors have been identified in observational and animal studies, and at present, they are only associated with changes in AD risk. Only further research, including clinical trials will reveal whether these factors can help to prevent AD. While more research is necessary, especially in the form of prevention trials, there is evidence showing a strong relationship between healthy ageing and a reduced risk of AD.

Our knowledge is growing rapidly as scientists expand their understanding of the many factors involved in the development of AD. Even though there are no treatments, drugs, or pills for curing AD, early identification and intervention are the best ways to delay/prevent and manage the disease. People can take some precautions that might reduce the effect of possible AD risk factors. These precautions include: lowering cholesterol and homocysteine levels, lowering high blood pressure levels, controlling diabetes, exercising regularly, and engaging in intellectually stimulating activities. It is advised to adopt a brain-healthy diet, keep physically and mentally active, and remain socially involved. All of these strategies are good to do anyway because they lower risk for other diseases and help maintain and improve overall health and well-being.

References

Adlard, P.A., V.M. Perreau, V. Pop and C.W. Cotman. 2005. "Voluntary exercise decreases amyloid load in a transgenic model of Alzheimer's disease". *J Neurosci.* 25: 4217–4221.

Alzheimer, A. 1907. "Uber eine eigenartige Erkankung der Hirnrinde". *Allg Psychiatrie* 64: 146–148.

Bagchi, K. (ed.), 2002. "Alzheimer's Disease in India". Society for Gerontological Research, New Delhi.

Bianchetti, A., R. Rozzini and M. Trabucchi. 2003. "Effects of acetyl-L-carnitine in Alzheimer's disease patients unresponsive to acetylcholinesterase inhibitors". *Curr Med Res Opin.* 19: 350–353.

Cole, G., G. Lim et al. 2001. "In India, the prevalence of Alzheimer's disease among 70 to 79 year olds is 4.4 fold less than that of the United States". *J Neuroscience* 21: 8370–8377.

Cole, G.M., T. Morihara, G.P. Lim, F. Yang, A. Begum and S.A. Frautschy. 2004. "NSAID and antioxidant prevention of Alzheimer's disease: Lessons from in vitro and animal models". *Ann N Y Acad Sci.* 1035: 68–84.

Fishel, M.A., G.S. Watson, T.J. Montine, Q. Wang, P.S. Green, J.J. Kulstad, D.G. Cook, E.R. Peskind, L.D. Baker, D. Goldgaber, W. Nie, S. Asthana, S.R. Plymate, M.W. Schwartz and S. Craft. 2005. "Hyperinsulinemia provokes synchronous increases in central inflammation and beta-amyloid in normal adults". *Arch Neurol* 62: 1539–1544.

Irizarry, M.C., M.E. Gurol, S. Raju, R. Diaz-Arrastia, J.J. Locascio, M. Tennis, B.T. Hyman, J.H. Growdon, S.M. Greenberg and T. Bottiglieri. 2005. "Association of homocysteine with plasma amyloid beta protein in aging and neurodegenerative disease". *Neurology* 65: 1402–1408.

Kivipelto, M., M.P. Laakso, J. Tuomilehto, A. Nissinen and H. Soininen. 2002. "Hypertension and hypercholesterolaemia as risk factors for Alzheimer's disease: Potential for pharmacological intervention". *CNS Drugs* 16: 435–444.

Kivipelto, M., A. Solomon and B. Winblad. 2005. "Statin therapy in Alzheimer's disease". *Lancet Neurol* 4: 521–522.

Lazarov, O., J. Robinson, Y.P. Tang, I.S. Hairston, Z. Korade-Mirnics, V.M. Lee, L.B. Hersh, R.M. Sapolsky, K. Mirnics and S.S. Sisodia. 2005. "Environmental enrichment reduces Abeta levels and amyloid deposition in transgenic mice". *Cell* 120: 701–713.

Lee, B.C.P., M. Mintun, R.L. Buckner and J.C. Morris. 2003. "Imaging of Alzheimer's Disease". *J Neuroimaging* 13: 199–214.

Lim, G.P., T. Chu, F. Yang, W. Beech, S.A. Frautschy and G.M. Cole. 2001. "The curry spice curcumin reduces oxidative damage and amyloid pathology in an Alzheimer transgenic mouse". *J Neurosci* 21: 8370–8377.

Oddo, S., L. Billings, P. Kesslak, D.H. Cribbs and F.M. LaFerla. 2004. "Aβ immunotherapy leads to clearance of early, but not late, hyperphosphorylated tau aggregates via the proteasome". *Neuron* 43: 321–332.

Ono, K., K. Hasegawa, H. Naiki and M. Yamada. 2005. "Curcumin has potent anti-amyloidogenic effects for Alzheimer's beta-amyloid fibrils in vitro". *J Neurosci Res.* 75: 742–750.

Ono, K., Y. Yoshiike, A. Takashima, K. Hasegawa, H. Naiki and M. Yamada. 2004. "Vitamin A exhibits potent antiamyloidogenic and fibril-destabilizing effects in vitro". *Exp Neurol* 189: 380–392.

Ravaglia, G., P. Forti, F. Maioli, M. Martelli, L. Servadei, N. Brunetti, E. Porcellini and F. Licastro. 2005. "Homocysteine and folate as risk factors for dementia and Alzheimer disease". *Am J Clin Nutr* 82: 636–643.

Reale, M., C. Iarlori, F. Gambi, I. Lucci, M. Salvatore and D. Gambi. 2005. "Acetylcholinesterase inhibitors effects on oncostatin-M, interleukin-1 beta and interleukin-6 release from lymphocytes of Alzheimer's disease patients". *Exp Gerontol.* 40: 165–171.

Rovio, S., I. Kareholt, E.L. Helkala, M. Viitanen, B. Winblad, J. Tuomilehto, H. Soininen, A. Nissinen and M. Kivipelto. 2005. "Leisure-time physical activity at midlife and the risk of dementia and Alzheimer's disease". *Lancet Neurol* 4: 705–711.

Shie, F.S., K.S. Montine, R.M. Breyer and T.J. Montine. 2005. "Microglial EP2 as a new target to increase amyloid beta phagocytosis and decrease amyloid beta-induced damage to neurons". *Brain Pathol.* 15: 134–138

Sjogren, M. and K. Blennow. 2005. "The link between cholesterol and Alzheimer's disease". *World J Biol Psychiatry* 6: 85–97.

Thakur, M.K. 2000. "Alzheimer's Disease: A challenge in the new millennium". *Curr Sci* 79: 101–108.

——. 2002. "Molecular studies in aging with special focus on Alzheimer's disease", in K. Bagchi (ed.), *Alzheimer's Disease in India*. Society of Gerontological Research, New Delhi, pp. 83–103.

Tucker, K.L., N. Qiao, T. Scott, I. Rosenberg and A. Spiro. 2005. "High homocysteine and low B vitamins predict cognitive decline in aging men: The veterans affairs normative aging study". *Am J Clin Nutr* 82: 627–635.

7 Mental Health

Roy Abraham Kallivayalil

> Mental illness is not a personal failure. It doesn't happen only to other people. There is no justification for excluding people with a mental illness or brain disorder from our communities – there is room for everyone. WHO is making a simple statement – mental health – neglected for far too long – is crucial to the overall well-being of individuals, societies and countries and must be universally regarded in a new light.
>
> —Dr Gro Harlem Brundtland (Director General, WHO, 2001)

We are in the new millennium and this should be a landmark in our understanding regarding the problems and difficulties of those who suffer from various forms of mental and psychological disorders. Attitudes must be challenged and new strategies put in place to minimize the negative impact mental health problems have on individual lives. In this context, older people deserve special mention and special consideration. The elderly face a greater likelihood of mental illness and they are an ever-increasing percentage of the population. The aetiology and clinical features of depression in old age, as well as other psychiatric disorders of old age, need to be understood in order to reduce their incidence and severity. Psychotherapy can play a role in mitigating the effects of mental illness. Reminiscence therapy can also be helpful. Medications are often effective but the use of them requires stringent supervision to prevent addiction and to ensure compliance. New models of collaboration and partnerships must be developed to maximize our effectiveness in improving quality of life for elderly citizens struggling with mental health issues.

Mental Health Policies

India has a rich, centuries-old heritage of medical and health sciences. The philosophy of Ayurveda and the surgical skills enunciated by Charaka and Shusharuta bear testimony to India's ancient tradition in the scientific health care of the people. The Constitution of India indicates the state's commitment to seeking to improve the health of its citizens. Establishment of a new social order based on equality, freedom, justice and the dignity of the individual, aiming at the elimination of poverty, ignorance and ill-health and directing the state to regard the raising the standard of living of its people and the improvement of public health as among its primary duties.

The Constitution of India

While this statement of commitment is encouraging, there is still practical work needed in order to help us achieve its goals. Over the centuries, with the intrusion of foreign influences and the mingling of cultures, various systems of medicine evolved and have continued to be practised widely. However, modern medicine has, in a relatively short period of time, made a major impact on the entire approach to health care and to the pattern of the development of health services infrastructure in the country.

Mental Health Policy in India: It is unfortunate that we still do not have a well-planned mental health policy in India. But it is a consolation that our health policy makes the following mention of mental health: Mental health must form an integral part of total health programme and as such should be included in all national policies and programmes in the field of health education and social welfare.

It may be worthwhile to have a bird's eye of our current health policy (2002):

- Mental health disorders are actually much more prevalent than is apparent on the surface.
- While such disorders do not contribute significantly to mortality, they have a serious bearing on the quality of life of the affected persons and their families.
- Mental health institutions are woefully deficient in physical infrastructure and trained manpower.
- NHP-2002 will address itself to these deficiencies in the public health sector.

- NHP-2002 envisages a network of decentralized mental health services for ameliorating the more common categories of disorders.
- The programme outline for such a disease would involve the diagnosis of common disorders, and the prescription of common therapeutic drugs, by general duty medical staff.
- In regard to mental health institutions for in-door treatment of patients, the policy envisages the upgrading of the physical infrastructure of such institutions at Central government expense so as to secure the human rights of this vulnerable segment of society.

It is imperative that all health activists rally around to support the formation of a new and coherent mental health policy for India. The health policy has been revised but there is at present no mental health policy. The National Mental Health Programme (1982) list objectives, and, in lieu of a newer and more detailed policy, this programme has been adopted and is currently used as the mental health policy in our country:

- Minimum mental health care for all (Particularly the most vulnerable and the under-privileged).
- To promote community participation.
- Integration of basic mental health care in general health care.
- Training primary health care personnel.
- Provision of neuro-psychiatric drugs in periphery.

Mental health financing in India is woefully inadequate as may be noted from the following facts: mental health care receives only 0.83 per cent of the total health care budget. There are some disability benefits for persons with mental disorders, but there is no comprehensive strategy for caring for those with mental health issues. In addition, there is not enough done to relieve the suffering of older people who have mental health problems. According to Mitchell Weiss (2001), "over the range of health priorities, mental health has been a neglected issue: failure to appreciate the nature of mental illness and the fact that much of it is treatable have contributed to this neglect".

An Ageing Society

India is one of the countries with the fastest growing number of older persons (those aged 65 years and above). China, India, and Indonesia are the three countries which are projected to have the largest number of older persons by the year 2025. In the last century, in India our life expectancy has considerably increased, making a significant transition in our demographic pattern. In 1901, India had 5 per cent of the population as older people, about 1.2 crores of people. This population has increased to 5.7 crores in 1990 and is expected to cross 10 crores by 2013. It is estimated that the elderly will constitute 21 per cent of the population by 2050. The elderly themselves are growing older, with people over the age of 80 years constituting a substantial number of the elderly population The current 80 million is three times Canada's total population.

It may be better to consider all those aged 65 years and more as older people (which is the norm in the West) although in India, we take 60 years to mark old age. In 1993, 6 per cent of world's population was over 65 years. This figure is an average of 14 per cent older people in developed countries and 4 per cent in less developed nations. Although the percentage of old people in less developed countries is smaller than in the developed nations, the absolute number of older people in the developing nations is quite high.

National Policy of Older People in India, 1999

- NGOs to make schemes for making elderly economically self-reliant.
- Providing routine screening for diseases.
- Tax incentives to encourage grown up children to look after aged parents.

We indeed have a national policy on older people declared in 1999, but it is hardly ever put into practice. While the National Policy of Older People in India is a good first step, progress toward the goals listed above is urgently needed.

Mental Health and the Elderly

Mental health of the elderly: Why is it important? The number of older persons will increase significantly all over the world and especially in the developing countries. This is all the more important in states like Kerala which has a very high life expectancy, almost as high as in the West. There is going to be a large number of older persons in such Indian States, and very little planning has been done by us so far. Many of the underlying factors which contribute to mental illness are preventable, and of those illnesses that are not preventable, many are treatable.

Effects of ageing on the brain: The ventricles in the brain enlarge and meninges thicken as we grow old. There will be decreased blood flow in the brain and decreased cortical grey matter (which can be seen in MRI scan). We loose brain weight as we grow older, 5 per cent between 30–70 years, 10 per cent by 70–80 years and 30 per cent by 90 years. But there is no cause for alarm, as well rehearsed skills like verbal comprehension, will be preserved. You may see that there is a balance between loss of flexible problem solving skills and the preserved benefits of accumulated wisdom.

Psychology of ageing: Several psychological changes occur due to ageing even in normal persons. There will be difficulty processing new information and there will be mental and physical slowing. Working memory will become poorer as evidenced by decreased performance, if attention has to be divided for two tasks. Older people may show the following emotional responses to stress: grief, guilt, loneliness; loss of meaning in life; lack of motivation; anxiety/anger/hostility; depression.

Personality traits of the aged: The personalities of the elderly are often marked by over cautiousness and rigidity. Generally, they will not be open to drastic changes. Physical health is also likely to decline and there may be some loss of sight or hearing or movement.

From the sociological perspective: There can be the stress of retirement and a consequent decline of income. Bereavement, widowhood, etc. may have to be faced. Illness in the elderly will be very stressful to the care givers. In India there have been societal changes which mean that the elderly have become unemployed (when, for example, agriculture became mechanized). The elderly have become increasingly dependent on younger people. There is often more social isolation among elderly people, although the problem is more pronounced in the West. In fact, 37 per cent of old people in UK live alone, whereas it is only 7 per cent in Chile, 3 per cent in China and less than 10 per cent in India.

Psychiatric Disorders in the Elderly

There is a wide range of psychiatric disorders. Physical illness increases vulnerability. Many illnesses are underestimated and undetected. Most psychiatric illnesses have an excellent prognosis with the correct intervention. Some of the most common psychiatric disorders in old age are depressive/mood disorders; later life delusional disorders; neurotic, stress related and somatoform disorders; personality disorders; alcoholism and drug abuse; disorders arising from abuse and neglect; Alzheimer's/vascular/other dementias; organic amnesic syndrome; delerium (non- alcoholic); organic hallucinosis, catatonic, delusional, organic mood disorders; and organic personality disorder.

Depression in Old Age

Depression remains the most common mental health problem among seniors. Its prevalence can be seen below. Prevalence: 3 per cent in community; 10 per cent in people above 65 years; 15 per cent in above 65 years in West; 75 per cent in institutionalized set up. While age is in itself not a risk factor, age brings with it, many vulnerabilities. Widowhood, chronic medical illness and somatic symptoms are all common in old age. There is a high rate of recurrence among individuals who suffer from late onset depression.

The aetiology of depression in old age is comprised of a combination of factors including the following: genetic (less significant); chronic disease and disability; dependent, anxious, avoidant personalities; stressful life-events; poor social support of old age depression. Clinical features; severe agitation and retardation (30%); cognitive impairment (60–70%). There appears to be no clear distinction of the clinical features of depression in the elderly compared with younger patients.

Clinical Features of Depression

Vulnerability to major depression with melancholic features are characterized by:

- Feelings of depression, hypochondriasis,
- Low self-esteem, feelings of worthlessness,
- Self-accusatory trends (sex, sinfulness)
- Paranoid and suicidal ideation
- Depressive delusions (poverty, physical illness)
- Nihilistic delusions ("Body is empty, non existent")
- Hallucinations (accusatory, obscene)
- Anxiety, hypochondriasis, confusion
- Masked depression

Depression: Course and Prognosis

The course and prognosis of depression is encouraging. With treatment 85 per cent of patients will improve considerably. Fifteen per cent of patients will not recover completely. The results of a three year follow up study show that one-third of patients were completely well; one-third of patients had recurrences and remissions; and the following one-third lived in a state of chronic invalidism. Depressions which have a good prognosis are those in patients with an onset before 70 years of age; those who have experienced a depression of a short duration and those with good PMP; those with no disabling physical illness; those who experience an earlier good recovery. Depressions with a bad prognosis include depressions in people with severe illness; those with poor drug compliance; those who have experienced stressful life events; and those with poorly adjusted personality.

The relationship between depression and physical illness remains strong. Illnesses associated with depression include the following: stroke, parkinson's disease, cancer, arthritis, cardiac disease, infections, and endocrine dysfunction. Any painful illnesses tend to increase depression.

There is also a relationship between depression and environment. Environmental factors can cause or worsen depression. The following factors influence depression: stressful life events, poor housing, poverty, social isolation, and unsatisfactory relationships. Depression in the elderly will require treatment following the same principles as are followed for the general public. Monitoring for suicidal feelings is crucial as the risk of suicide is higher in people suffering from depression. Antidepressants can be utilized but should be prescribed with caution. It is important to note that medicine compliance is not good in the depressed population. There is a tendency toward over- or under-medicating. Doctors will need to treat any co-morbidity.

Psychotherapy for depressed seniors can be useful. Support and encouragement are needed. The patient needs to know that depression is an illness, not moral failure. Supportive/interpersonal/cognitive/ Reminiscence therapies can all play a role. Counselling of spouse and/or family is often useful. Psychotherapy should be made available as it helps to relieve tensions and it enables seniors to work within their functional status. The result of psychotherapy is improved memory, greater mental alertness, improved gait, and less urinary incontinence. Therapists can be active, supportive and flexible.

Older people seek therapy to enjoy their therapist's unqualified and unlimited support. They often seek reassurance and approval. The therapist may be seen as "all powerful, all knowing", leading the patient to expect a magical cure, whereas in fact a collaborative effort is required. Reminiscence (life review) therapy is another form of therapy that can be successful. Using the universal tendency of the ageing person to reflect or reminisce about past meaningful or conflictual memories, reminiscence therapy encourages older patients to resolve issues and remember positive events. The therapy encourages a reunion with family, good friends, books, and albums. Life review therapy often increases tolerance to conflicts, relieves the elderly of guilt and fear, enhances their self-esteem, creativity, and acceptance. Late-life depression appears to be the exception as it does not always respond to life review therapies as well as depression in early or mid life. There is a tendency to chronicity and relapse. Late-life depression is associated with poor physical health. Only 20 per cent of those who experience late-life depression remain well for more than five years afterward. One-third of those who suffer have persistent depressive symptoms. Mortality may be higher. Prognosis improves with appropriate treatment. Depression is not an unavoidable consequence of old age and it is recognizable and treatable. Anti-depressants and psychotherapy may be superior forms of treatment.

Personality disorders make up a sizable proportion of the mental health cases. Social isolation for those with paranoid traits can be a challenge. Senile squalor syndrome causes seniors to be isolated, filthy and to neglect themselves.

Alcoholism and drug abuse are also mental health issues faced by the elderly. Alcoholism can be of recent onset or can be of longer term. Drug abuse often causes problems for older people, in particular, hypnotics, laxatives, and analgesics cause addictions. Some addictions are caused inadvertently when the older person takes a medication to relieve a medical symptom and continues too long, causing the addition, or the older person knowingly continues a medication because they enjoy or believe they need the feeling it gives them.

Dementia in the Elderly

It may not be easy to diagnose dementia in the very early stages. It may be mistaken for normal changes of ageing, or poor intelligence, or merely as lack of education. But the correct diagnosis is of paramount importance and, when in doubt, the opinion of an expert must be obtained. The prevalence of dementia rises steeply with age. Alzheimer's type dementia is more common in Europe, North America and Australia, while vascular dementia is more common in the Far East.

Alzheimer's disease (or Alzheimer's dementia or AD) is the most common form of dementia in the elderly. The prevalence rate for the moderate and severe forms is 2–7 per cent in people who are 65 years and above. Mild forms are excluded from this statistic due to difficulty in diagnosis. Alzheimer's disease is rare before 60 years. How do you recognize Alzheimer's disease? The first evidence is usually minor forgetfulness. Gradually, it increases during the next 2–4 years leading to increased memory loss and lack of spontaneity. Language will be affected and they will have difficulty to find the suitable word or the name for objects. There may be disorientation in time. They will find it very difficult to cope in unfamiliar places eg: when on a holiday. The mood may be depressed in the majority of cases. Hallucinations occur in the late stages. Due to forgetfulness, they may develop delusions and say their belongings have been stolen by others. Their behaviour is often disturbed. They may be restless or they may wake up at night perplexed and disoriented. The sleep-wake schedule may be disrupted. Sometimes they become aggressive – verbally and physically. They may wander about and over-eat or under-eat. Their self-care will be poor and social behaviour may be inappropriate. Many people may maintain a façade of normality especially in the early stages, which might mislead the family into thinking that there is nothing seriously wrong.

New treatments are now emerging for this illness. It is believed that the neurotransmitter level especially of Acetyl Choline goes down in AD. Hence, new drugs – Acetyl Choline estrase inhibitors like Donepezil are increasingly used in the treatment of AD. But no treatment has yet been discovered to arrest or reverse the dementing disease process. Psychological and social treatments are also essential. The patient and the family should be helped to cope with the illness. Encouragement, support, help and understanding are needed. Caring for the carers is also important.

Barriers to Care

There are several socio-cultural barriers to accepting the right psychiatric or physical treatment. The most common barriers are:

- Influence of culture/values
- Non-acceptance of psychiatric or psychological service
- Medical treatment of somatic or bodily illnesses (without recognising that they may be psychological in origin)
- Seeking non-professionals/healers
- Underestimation of mental health needs

Our society also has a tendency to deny mental health needs. The following are the main reasons:

- These problems are shameful.
- Mental health may be a punishment for misdeeds.

- There is a prevailing sentiment that "suffering should be endured".
- Emotional control is valued in society.
- Seeking help indicates that one is "not in control".

Some of the problems facing the developing nations in the care of the elderly include the following: poor facilities, poor funding, lack of staff caused by 'brain-drain' resulting in huge clinical case-loads, little time for mental health research, and a general sense of mental health issues being a low priority.

Some of the advantages that India has include the following: elders wield power due to wealth; elders are cared for by younger citizens as a duty; in India no payment is given for caring for an elderly relative; social isolation is not a major problem, just 5 per cent of the elderly in India live alone compared to 37 per cent in UK and USA; the role of spirituality; and the role of the family all mitigate against the enormous challenges faced by mental health providers and their clients.

Future Plans – New Models

One of the goals shared among many mental health professionals is to participate in collaborative research with western colleagues. Though at present the huge burden of illness and several other constraints present challenges to such partnerships, they are still seen as valuable and worthy of serious effort. Another goal is to establish global databases and networks and to involve researchers from low income countries in discussions and projects. The model centres on the sharing of knowledge in order to learn as much as possible about mental health issues for the elderly and to determine the best practices for treating them. Several agencies are attempting to encourage collaboration. They include the Indian Psychiatric Society (Geriatric Psychiatric Section), The Association of Physicians of India, The Geriatric Society of India, The Alzheimer's and Related Disorders Society of India (ARDSI) and other NGOs, and university departments. Most of these organizations lack adequate funding and official support or patronage. So we have miles to go in this regard.

New Models of Collaboration – Principles

- Mutual trust and shared decision making
- National ownership
- Putting research findings into policy and practice
- Development of national research capacity

Future Plans – Partnership

- Partnership in research
- Organizing community care services for the elderly
- Health education
- Public awareness through media
- Publication of data
- Training programmes/exchanges for faculty/PG trainees

The Need for Partnership

World Mental Health Report (Dejarlais et al., 1995) and the Global Burden of disease study (Murray and Lopez, 1996) draws attention to developing countries. Sensitizing, training, and equipping rural and urban health centres is of the utmost importance. In developing countries there is a huge burden of illness, severe disability in mental illness, and very few mental health research networks or centres (Jablensky 1999).

Conclusion

The mental health of the elderly is a grossly neglected area in India. We are now facing a huge increase in the number of older persons with the increase in life expectancy. We need a comprehensive plan to deal with this crisis situation. Governments should take the lead in this matter. Professional organizations, social activists, NGOs and spirited members of the public should come together and make the lives of our older persons happy and productive. It is our responsibility towards ourselves. We need a concrete mental health policy and we need actions to complement the statements made in our policies. Mental health professionals need to share knowledge regarding depression, dementia, and disease in order to find improved ways of treating them. New models for partnerships with western colleagues need to be developed to encourage the mobilization of knowledge.

References

Ezra, H.F. et al. 2003. "Introduction to Cultural Psychiatry" in *Textbook of Clinical Psychiatry*, 4th ed., R.E. Hales and S.C. Yudofsky (eds.), Washington DC: American Psychiatric Publishing.

Levenson, James L. 2005. *Textbook of Psychosomatic Medicine*. Washington DC: American Psychiatric Publishing.

Vaccaro, J.V. 2000. *Managed Care: Comprehensive Text Book of Psychiatry*. 7th ed., B.J. Sadock and V.A. Sadock (eds.), Philadelphia: Lippincott, Williams and Wilkins.

Weiss, Mitchell G. 2001. "Global, National, and Local Approaches to Mental Health: Examples from India". *Tropical Medicine and International Health*, VI: 1.

WHO. 2001. "Atlas: Country Profiles on Mental Health Resources". Geneva.

Wig, N.N. 1983. "DSM III: A Perspective from the Third World", in R.L. Spitzer, J.B.W. Williams and A.E. Skodel (eds.), *International Perspectives of DSM III*. Washington DC: American Psychiatric Press Inc.

8 Health Promotion and Protection

B. Krishnaswamy and G.S. Shanthi

Ageing has become a global concern as the percentage of the elderly population is increasing rapidly. The implications of an ageing population for individuals, family, communities, and the country are going to be enormous, especially in developing countries like India. Rapid rise of ageing population relates epidemiologically to an increasing prevalence of chronic diseases and disability. From a social aspect, a greater number of the elderly will require formal services, as the traditional social structures are eroding.

From the public health perspective, the goal is to keep people alive and healthy as long as possible; hence emphasis is now laid on the functional status of the elderly and on the concept of 'successful ageing'. Successful ageing is used to describe individuals who do not exhibit age-related declines in physiologic and metabolic variables. 'normal ageing' is related to age associated decline in functional capacity and 'impaired ageing' is related to a diseased state. To maintain the elderly in good health, good mobility and independent functional status, health education and health promotion play a very important role. Health is defined by the WHO as a state of complete physical, mental and social well-being, which is not merely an absence of disease or infirmity, but also an ability to lead a socially and economically productive life.

This is an idealistic goal rather than a realistic proposition. The WHO study group devised an 'operational definition' which states that health is a condition or quality of a human organism, expressing the adequate functioning of the organism in given conditions, including genetic or environmental. In a society, a 'health care system' is an important determinant of health.

Optimal health in old age means:

- freedom from illness,
- optimal functional status,
- adequate system of social support, and
- continuing personal development

Figure 8.1 ***Health Care – Illness Care (Treatment and Rehabilitation)***

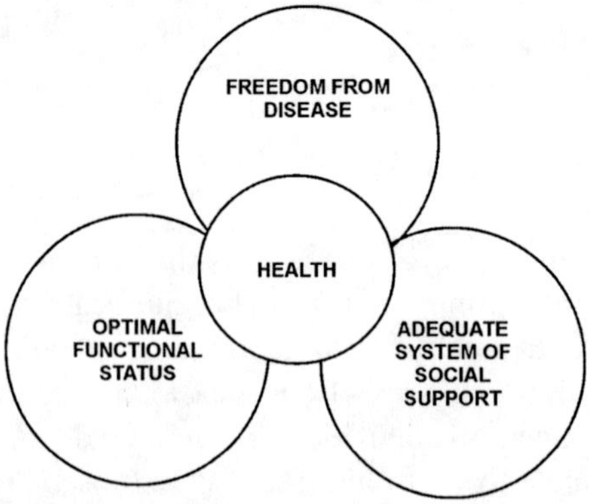

Preventive Health Care

Levels of prevention are as follows:

1. Primordial prevention	Prevention of development of risk factors.
2. Primary prevention	Action taken prior to the onset of disease by elimination or modification of the risk factors.
3. Secondary prevention	Helps to halt the progress of disease and prevent complications.
4. Tertiary prevention	Intervention in the late pathogenesis stage.

Health Promotion

The WHO (1986) had defined health promotion as "the process of enabling people to increase control over and to improve their health". This is primary prevention.

Reasons for Health Promotion of the Elderly

1. Prevents or delays the onset of risk factors of disease.
2. Prevents the onset of full-blown disease and its complications.
3. Decreases the morbidity and maintains the quality of life.
4. Helps to maintain the independence and functional status of the elders.

5. Prevents social and economic burdens for society.
6. While primary ageing (genetically determined) is inevitable, secondary ageing (due to avoidable and preventable diseases) can be diminished to zero, making the concept of "compression of morbidity" viable, i.e., rendering the period of sickness, disability and dependency squeezed into a brief period just before death.

These reasons support "successful ageing' which should be the goal of every senior citizen. Successful ageing is a combination of physical health, mental health, psychosocial adjustment and life satisfaction.

Health Literacy

Health education is important in bringing about lifestyle modifications, and safe medication usage, and in implementing rehabilitation measures. Improved esteem and self-worth can empower the elderly person to have the confidence to become more health literate. A multidimensional strategy for ensuring health and well-being in old age is as follows:

Figure 8.2 ***A Multi-dimensional Strategy for Well-being in Old Age***

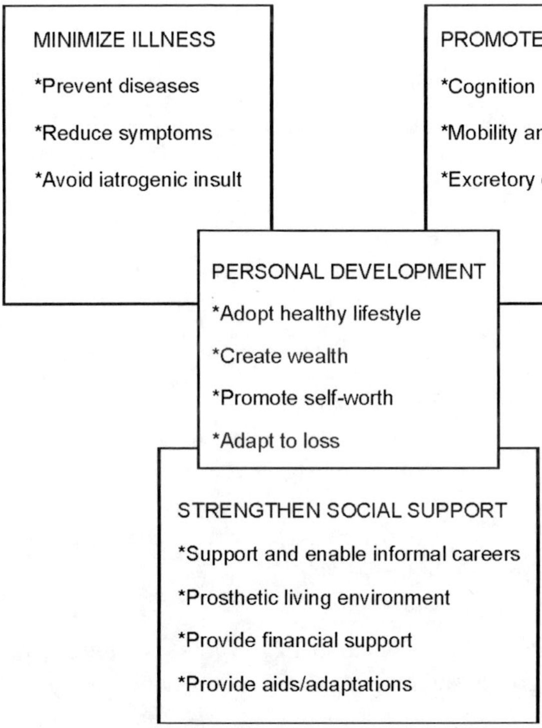

Clinical Preventive Health Care

Primary Prevention		*Secondary Prevention*	
Counselling and lifestyle modification	Tobacco avoidance, Nutrition, regular exercise, safe driving, estrogen replacement	Early detection	Hypertension (B.P measurement) Coronary artery disease (serum lipid test)
Vaccinations	Influenza Pneumoccous Tetanus	Screening for malignancies	Breast cancer (Mammography) Cervical cancer (Cervical smear) Colorectal carcinoma (Fecal occult blood test)
		Special senses	Visual loss (Sight card) Hearing loss (Whisper test or audioscope)
		Miscellaneous	Problem drinking, Injury prevention

Counselling About Lifestyle Modification

Tobacco

Smoking is the most important and potentially reversible risk factor for many diseases. Some related diseases are:

1. Vascular	Coronary artery disease Hypertension Myocardial infarction and sudden death Cerebrovascular accidents Ischaemic peripheral vascular disease
2. Pulmonary	Bronchitis Emphysema Pneumonia Chronic obstructive pulmonary disease
3. Malignancies	Bronchogenic carcinoma Cancer of oral cavity, pharynx, esophagus and stomach Carcinoma of bladder

Studies of the elderly population have shown significant benefit from implementing quit-smoking strategies. Clinicians should actively discourage elders from smoking. It improves the quality of life and longevity of the individual and also benefits society (reduces the risk of passive smoking).

Nutrition

Nutrition, health and ageing are inextricably linked. Proper nutrition as a part of an active, healthy lifestyle is a key to successful ageing. Diet modification helps in disease prevention.

Saturated fats avoided	CAHD Dyslipidemias Carcinoma of colon
Sodium restriction	Hypertension
Calorie restriction	Maintains body weight Elderly male and female: 1600–3000 kcal according to their activity

Anti-ageing is measured by

1. Prevention of age-related functional deterioration
2. Retardation of onset of age-related disease
3. Extension of mean and maximum life spans

High fiber diet (20 gm/day)	Diverticular disease of colon Colonic malignancy Constipation
Calcium (1200–1500 mg/day)	Osteoporosis
Vitamins	
β-carotene	Malignancies
Folate	Vascular disease (homocystinemia) Colorectal malignancy

Reasons for Poor Nutrition in the Elderly

1. Poor dentition
2. Dysphagia
3. Comorbid conditions
4. Depression, dementia
5. Loneliness
6. Alcoholism

Consequences of Undernutrition

1. Frailty
2. Physical dependence

3. Premature death
4. Impairment of immune system
5. Increased risk of infection
6. Poor wound healing

Exercise

In old age there is an inevitable functional decline leading to functional dependency. Surveys show that by age 75 one in three men and one in two women are not physically active. In the elderly, exercise increases physical fitness. This helps older adults to improve, maintain or regain the functional status needed to perform activities of daily living (ADL) and instrumental activities of daily living (IADL) which contribute to 'quality of life'.

Benefits of Exercise

1. Promotes a sense of well-being
2. Increases cardiorespiratory capacity
3. Improves muscle strength
4. Increases endurance
5. Increases bone mass
6. Maintains flexibility
7. Increases the range of motion in joints
8. Increases lean body mass
9. Improves balance – prevention of falls and fractures
10. Improves sleep

Types of Exercises Recommended

The National Institute of Health recommends four types of exercises for the well-being of the elderly:

(i) *Strengthening exercise:* Builds muscle as well as increases metabolism, which helps to keep the blood sugar and weight under control.

(ii) *Balance exercise:* Helps build leg muscles and prevent falls. These exercises help to maintain independence and avoid disabilities that may result from falling.

(iii) *Stretching exercise:* Gives more freedom of movement. Range of movement exercises in hospitalized patients help to prevent contractures.

(iv) *Endurance exercises:* Walking, jogging, and swimming increase the heart rate and breathing for an extended period of time, and build up endurance gradually.

Types of Exercise Avoided

Isometric exercises should be avoided as they increase blood pressure and cardiac workload.

Contraindications for Exercise

1. Aortic stenosis
2. Severe congestive heart failure
3. HOCM
4. Uncontrolled hypertension

With regular exercise and good nutrition, obesity is avoided, which is a risk factor for many diseases. Regular physical activity protects against osteoporosis, non-insulin dependent diabetes mellitus, hypertension, ischaemic heart disease and stroke. Also, there is evidence to support the value of exercise for fall prevention. People who are at high risk for falls should be offered a programme of exercise incorporating muscle strengthening and balance training (e.g., Tai Chi).

Safe Driving

The risk of motor vehicle injuries increases with the age of the driver (after middle age). Hence counselling, regarding primary disease, (neurological, syncope, DM, arthritis, vision defects) avoidance of alcohol, timing of drugs (psychoactive drugs), use of seat belts for all journeys, is needed.

Estrogen Replacement

Based on the results of various studies, postmenopausal women are advised to have hormone replacement therapy (HRT).

Benefits of HRT

1. Decreases cardiovascular diseases.
2. Prevents osteoporosis and fractures of hip, vertebrae and wrist.
3. Prevents Alzheimer's disease.

4. Suppresses menopausal symptoms.
5. Increases sense of well-being.

Risks of HRT

1. Breast cancer
2. Uterine body cancer

Detailed history and regular screening is advised before commencing HRT.

Vaccination

Influenza vaccine	All people >65 years should have an annual vaccination of strain specific influenza vaccine.
Pneumococcal vaccine	All people of >65 years should be vaccinated once with a 23-valent preparation. High-risk patients should be revaccinated after six years (Dialysis patients and asplenic patients).

Indications for Pneumococcal and Influenza Vaccine

1. Institutionalized elderly
2. COPD
3. Diabetes mellitus
4. Chronic renal failure
5. Nephrotic syndrome
6. Congestive cardiac failure
7. Ischaemic heart disease
8. Cirrhosis of liver

Tetanus Inoculation

Tetanus is less common in the elderly but has a high likelihood of fatality. Inoculation is recommended every 10 years in view of higher risk of accidents and injuries in old age. A single booster vaccination at the age of 65 years is routinely advised.

Contraindications of Vaccination

1. Severe allergic reaction.
2. Anaphylactic reaction to eggs.
3. H/o. Guillain barre or other neurologic syndromes after influenza vaccine.

Secondary Prevention

Aims

To prevent disability by early detection of sub-clinical cases through screening or case finding. The common causes of morbidity and mortality are:

1. Cardiovascular diseases
2. Cerebrovascular diseases
3. Malignancies

Screening is Recommended by US Preventive Services Task Force 1995 and Canadian Task Force

1. Blood pressure
2. Height and weight
3. Serum lipid measurement
4. Fecal occult blood (annually) and/or sigmoidoscopy
5. Mammography and clinical breast examination (every 1–2 years)
6. Papinocaloau test (all women who are/have been sexually active with an intact cervix)
7. Vision screening
8. Assessment for hearing impairment
9. Assessment of potential problem drinking

Hypertension

- Prevalence > 70 per cent in elderly.
- Both systolic and diastolic hypertension, are associated with cardiovascular and cerebrovascular diseases.
- Several trials like STOP (Swedish trial of older patients with hypertension) SHEP (Systolic hypertension in elderly people), MRC (Medical Research Council) have proved that the treatment of hypertension is beneficial as a means of substantially reducing stroke, cardiac events and death.

Screening for Malignancies

Screening is warranted in the elderly, as the incidence of malignancy increases with age. The reasons are as follows:

1. Decline in immune function – decrease T cell mediated immunity and IL-2 response.
2. Prolonged environmental exposures to carcinogens.

3. Physiologic changes like:
   (a) Abnormal DNA transcription, proof reading and repair
   (b) Alteration in metabolic clearance of toxins

Carcinoma Breast

It is the most common malignancy in women. Between 50–69 years, clinical examination of the breast and a mammography are recommended annually. In women >75 years an annual physical examination of the breasts alone is advised except in people with (a) Family history of breast cancer and (b) Carcinoma of contralateral breast. Several trials demonstrated survival benefits for screened people.

Carcinoma Cervix

Even though it is a disease of young women, 1/4th of new cases occur after the age of 65 years. Hence screening is continued up to 65 years, which has reduced the incidence of invasive disease. If repeated screening results are persistently normal, screening can be discontinued after the age of 65 years.

Carcinoma Colon

The incidence rises steeply with ageing in both sexes. Early detection and treatment improves the outcome. Annual faecal occult blood testing is recommended as sigmoidoscopy and colonoscopy are relatively expensive, and require expert physician care. Adequate preparation of the elderly is difficult. Relative insensitivity is the drawback. Hence colonoscopy is recommended once in every five years and sigmoidoscopy once in every 3–5 years.

Indications for Colonoscopy

- Familial adenomatous polyposis.
- Hereditary nonpolyposis colon cancer.

Screening for Special Senses

Vision

Reduced visual acuity in the elderly may be due to

1. Presbyopia
2. Cataracts
3. Open angle glaucoma
4. Macular degeneration
5. Diabetic retinopathy

Screening is done using Snellen's Chart and regular fundus examination.

Hearing Loss

One third of older people are unaware of their disability. Regular screening is essential. Screening is done by (i) Whisper test (sensitive, inexpensive) and (ii) Audioscope.

Counselling is done to avoid excessive noise and ototoxic drugs. Use of hearing aids is advised.

Alcohol Consumption

Excessive alcohol consumption is hazardous, while modest intake (1 to 2 drinks per day) is beneficial). Problem drinking precedes serious alcoholism and is amenable to counselling. Problem drinking is detected by questionnaires like CAGE questions.

Injury Prevention

Injuries, particularly falls, are an important cause of death in the elderly. Intrinsic risk factors lead to recurrent falls. Falls prevention strategies involving increase of muscle strength, endurance and balances improve the functional status, and have been proven useful in a large multicentric research FISCIT (Frailty and Injuries Co-operative of Intervention Techniques).

Atrial Fibrillation

It is a common cardiac arrhythmia of old age. The most important risk is embolic stroke (5% per year). Hence anticoagulation is advised.

Recurrent M.I. and Stroke

Secondary prevention also denotes prevention of recurrent illness like M.I. and stroke. Use of Aspirin and β blockers in M.I patients and aspirin/antiplatelets, antihypertensives in stroke patients reduce the risk of recurrent episodes.

Tertiary Prevention

Tertiary prevention is defined as the prevention of morbidity or mortality from established disease, by disability limitation, and rehabilitation.

In Geriatric medicine, the common indications are:

1. Rehabilitation following hip fracture.
2. Stroke rehabilitation by multidisciplinary intervention.

3. Arthritis relief by medications and exercise.
4. Osteoporosis detection before a disability fracture occurs.
5. Vascular disease (coronary, cerebral and peripheral) occurs due to risk factors like hypertension, smoking, diabetes, atrial fibrillation and dyslipidemia. Treatment of vascular risk factors significantly reduces subsequent stroke, MI, or limb loss.

This chronic disease management is based on expert guidelines and practice-based protocols for specific illnesses.

Additional Disease Prevention Activities in Selected Elderly People

Prostatic Malignancy

Prostatic malignancy is a common cancer in older males. Prostate specific antigen (PSA) concentrations correlate directly with age. The rise is 0.04ng/ml/year, which is due to typical increase in prostate volume of 0.5ml/year. It is a specific tumour marker for men >60 years of age.

Screening is done by: (1) Digital rectal examination but it is insensitive, (2) PSA assessment is highly sensitive but has low predictive value. (3) USG assessment of prostate to assess the prostate size, volume and contour (non-invasive test) (4) Biopsy of the prostate is the confirmative test.

Asymptomatics do not benefit from early treatment. Therefore screening remains controversial.

Diabetic Complications

Some experts recommend screening obese persons. Blood glucose testing is recommended every 1–3 years, as older adults have significant risk of retinopathy, nephropathy, and coronary disease.

Cognitive Impairment

As most cognitive abilities decline with age, the clinicians should follow-up the symptoms of cognitive loss. Early minimal cognitive impairment (MCI) should be detected and periodic screening must be done to identify dementia.

Depression

Depression is a common problem in the elderly. It increases their mortality rate. Untreated depression is associated with both psychiatric and general medical consequences. In the treatment for depression, selective serotonin reuptake inhibitors (SSRI) are commonly used followed by tricyclic antidepressants (TCA) and others. However screening does not show significant benefits.

Osteoporosis

The morbidity due to osteoporosis warrants early detection. The availability of noninvasive and gold standard tests of bone mineral density to detect osteoporosis in the asymptomatic stage has made diagnosising easy. However it is expensive and hence recommended mainly in asymptomatic women with multiple osteoporosis risk factors or in men and women with chronic glucocorticoid use.

Hypothyroidism

Some experts recommend screening women, as hypothyroidism is prevalent among them. Yearly estimation of thyrotrophin hormone can detect the disease in a preclinical stage.

Screening for Frailty

Frailty is due to a breakdown in the dynamic balance between the individual's strengths and deficits. Deficits in physical and cognitive functioning threaten the autonomy of individuals. The prevalence of frailty rises with age due to the presence of chronic disabilities. Factors, which predict the onset of frailty, are self-perception of health, various diseases (stroke, osteoarthritis, hip fracture) mental abilities and physical factors like muscular strength and endurance. Tests of functional decline include the following: timed manual performance of activities; lower limb performance such as standing balance; five repetitions of rising from a chair and sitting down, etc.

It is not yet known whether screening for frailty or potential frailty and targeted interventions will prevent the onset of frailty and disability. This requires further research.

Health Promotion Programmes

1. Health promotion programmes are developed using evidence-based strategies and therefore are cost-effective.
2. They provide data on the health status and health behaviours of older adults, to help monitor health trends and outcomes.
3. They expand communication efforts to promote healthy lifestyles among older adults.
4. Programmes of "true health promotion" reduce cost.

Conclusion

The health of the community depends on the lifestyle (physical activity, nutrition, mental stimulation, smoking and alcohol), safe environment, social support and a regular health care system. Health promotion and protection is a combined effort involving health care workers, planners, politicians and the senior citizen themselves.

Bibliography

Canadian Task Force on the Periodic Health Examination: "Canadian Guide to Clinical Preventive Health Care". 1994. Canadian Communication Group, Ottawa.

Cumming, R.G. 1990. "Calcium intake and bone mass: A quantitative review of the evidence". *Calcified Tissue International* 47, pp. 194–201.

Eddy, D.M. 1989. "Screening for Breast Cancer". *Annals of Internal Medicine* 111, pp. 389–99.

Fiatarone, M.A., E.F. O'Neill, N.D. Ryan et al. 1994. "Exercise training and nutritional supplementation for physical frailty in very old people". *New England Journal of Medicine* 330, pp. 1769–75.

Kaplan, G.A., W.J. Strawbridge, T. Camocho and R.D. Cohen. 1993. "Factors associated with change in physical functioning in the elderly: A 6-year prospective study". *Journal of Aging and Health* 5, pp. 140–53.

Lacroix, A.Z. and G.S. Omen. 1992. "Older adults and smoking". *Clinics in Geriatric Medicine* 8, pp. 69–87.

Lindsay, R. 1987. "Estrogen therapy in the prevention and management of osteoporosis". *American Journal of Obstetrics and Gynecology* 156, pp. 1347–56.

Reuben, D.B., T.T. Yoshikawa and R.W. Besdine (eds.), 1993. *Geriatrics Review Syllabus Supplement*. 3rd ed., American Geriatrics Society, New York, p. 172.

Tinneti, M.E., D.I. Baker, G. McAvay et al. 1994. "A multifactorial intervention to reduce the risk of falling among elderly people living in the community". *New England Journal of Medicine* 331, pp. 821–7.

US Preventive Services Task Force. 1989 and 1996. *Guide to Clinical Preventive Services*. 1st and 2nd editions. Williams and Wilkins, Baltimore.

9 Physical Activity and Ageing

Gareth R. Jones and C. Shanthi Johnson

Physical activity and exercise have been long established as means of mitigating the potential burden of an ageing population, though not only disease prevention, but even more importantly, through the preservation of physiological reserve capacity or fitness. Continued physical activity allows older adults to continue to perform many tasks of daily living, required for independent function, even in the face of compounding disease and/or disability. Nevertheless, older adults typically become more sedentary. Their ability to perform activities becomes more limited as a result of the compounding affect of chronic disease and physiological deterioration. Arguably, increased inactivity may be the result of pressure directed toward older adults to conform to societal pressures and inadequate information on the benefits and importance of daily exercise in preserving functional independence in old age. This chapter will draw attention to new perspectives regarding the dose of physical activity required to help prevent disease, and more significantly, to maintain independent function in old age.

What is the Message?

Active living, physical activity, exercise and fitness are often used collectively throughout the academic literature as a panacea for disease prevention and in the case of older adults as a means of mitigating the functional losses experienced with growing old. Unfortunately, in most cases, they are often used inappropriately. For example, health advocacy groups promote the importance of general leisure activity, such as, housework, casual recreational activities walking, bowling, and painting, may actually confer increased fitness or at least improved health. This perception is based on epidemiological data related to cardiovascular disease and all-cause mortality, where leisure activity of moderate-vigorous intensity appears to be protective (Morris et al., 1980; Paffenbarger et al., 1986). However, for older adults, only higher intensity physical activity (activity verging on exercise) is truly related to a reduction in cardiovascular risk and poor fitness, while physical activity *per se* is responsible for increased all-cause mortality risk in seniors (Blair et al., 1989, 1995). However, before we can fully understand the issues regarding appropriate health promotion strategies, one must first understand what the terminology actually means.

Active living is a way of life where people choose to be physically active every day in their community; whether they are at school, at work, at home, or at play. It may involve both structured (sports) and unstructured (play) activities.

Physical activity is defined as any bodily movement produced by skeletal muscle that results in energy expenditure.

Exercise, a subset of physical activity, which is a planned, structured, repetitive bodily movement done to improve one or more of the components of fitness.

Fitness is a set of attributes that people have or achieve relating to their ability to perform physical activity. These attributes have traditionally included cardiorespiratory function, muscular strength, body composition, flexibility, and, more recently, balance skills have been accepted as a component of fitness in older adults. Nevertheless, this terminology is often diluted for public consumption where both scientists and health advocates sugarcoat the exercise dose message with holistic ideals such as active living.

To put this into perspective one must only review public health recommendations made over the past 25 years in regards to the amount and type of physical activity and/or exercise needed to confer health benefits. During the 1970s, the American College of Sports Medicine (ACSM), the American Heart Association (AHA), and other national organizations began issuing physical activity recommendations to the public on the beneficial effects of vigorous exercise on cardiorespiratory fitness. These recommendations generally focused on cardiorespiratory endurance and specified sustained periods of vigorous physical activity involving large muscle groups and lasting at least 20 minutes on 3 or more days per week. As understanding of the benefits of less vigorous activity grew, recommendations followed suit. During the past few years, the ACSM, the AHA, the Centre's for Disease Control (CDC), and the National Institute of Health (NIH) have all recommended regular, moderate-intensity physical activity as an option for those who get little or no exercise. More recent evidence from the Institute of Medicine (Brooks et al., 2005) now suggests that 60–90 minutes of moderate activity is required most days of the week. The evolution of these guidelines suggests an emerging relationship between the health advocates' recommendation and the North American population that is ageing rapidly and getting fatter exponentially.

Underpinning these recommendations is a growing understanding of how physical activity affects physiological function. The bodies of both young and old respond to exercise in ways that have important positive effects on musculoskeletal, cardiovascular, respiratory, and endocrine systems. These changes are consistent with a number of health benefits, including a reduced risk of premature mortality and reduced risks of coronary heart disease, hypertension, colon cancer, and diabetes mellitus. Regular participation in physical activity also appears to reduce depression and anxiety, improve mood, and enhance ability to perform daily tasks throughout the lifespan. This message is most important to older adults where independent lifestyle, regardless of age-associated morbidity, is of paramount concern. However, questions remain regarding the amount and type, as well as the intensity and frequency of physical activity required to preserve the functional independence of seniors.

Cardiorespiratory Fitness

Normal age-related changes in cardiorespiratory fitness, musculoskeletal strength and body composition directly contribute to reducing individual physiological reserve capacity of many older adults. Although physiological reserve capacity is not precisely defined, many older people live perilously close to important functional thresholds required for independent daily living, needing only a minor illness or disabling event to render them dependent. Dependence and associated reductions to quality of life is of concern to older adults and a financial burden to the health care system. Although frailty and dependence may result in the loss of physical function, improvement or at least maintenance of cardiorespiratory fitness is seen as one intervention that may reduce the years of dependent living, and improve the quality of life of older adults.

Both young and old can enjoy the health benefits of aerobic exercise, yet older adults may have the most to gain from maintaining and/or improving their aerobic fitness. An individual's aerobic fitness indicates their ability to perform physical activity lasting two minutes or longer. Recent research shows that after accounting for the effect of diseases, poor aerobic fitness is directly responsible for increased morbidity and premature mortality in older adults (Franco et al., 2005; Paterson et al., 2004)

Morey and his colleagues (1998) provided an important contribution to the understanding of fitness, especially cardiorespiratory fitness, by identifying the functional limitations of older adults. Their model (Figure 9.1) indicates the causes of functional limitations (etiology of disability) whereby a lack of cardiorespiratory fitness ($\dot{V}O_2max$), muscle strength, and morphology (including body composition, flexibility and bone density) produce a potential limitation of function in older adults. Other social-demographic and behavioral factors (age, education, depression, body-mass index) were controlled for as confounders. Their sample of older (average 72.5 years) men and women included those with a variety of chronic health conditions (arthritis, cardiovascular disease, orthopaedic problems), and symptoms (pain, shortness of breath, memory loss). Results showed that factors other than pathology lead to functional limitations. In fact all three fitness components were significantly associated with loss of function. Therefore, lack of fitness was an impairment, and important critical modifier in the path to disability. Further, cardiorespiratory fitness was directly associated with pathology, but even more importantly with functional limitations independent of pathology. These authors conclude that cardiorespiratory fitness is important in preventing cardiovascular disease and all cause-mortality, and exercise training (cardiorespiratory and muscular performance) is important as a means to attenuate functional decline.

Figure 9.1 ***Contribution of Fitness to Becoming Functionally Dependent in Later Life***

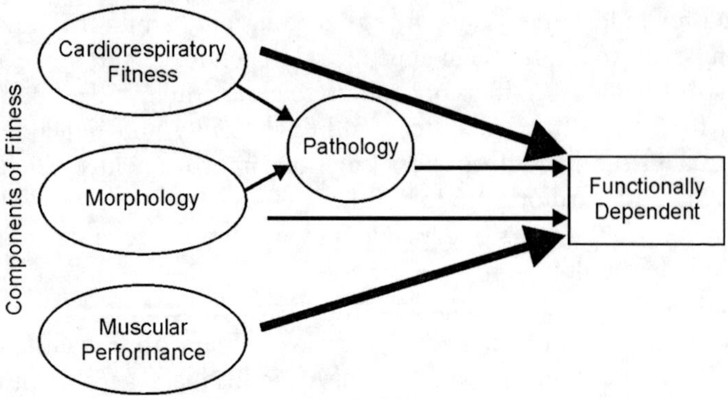

(Adapted from Morey et al., 1998)

Those who are sedentary can expect to experience a 16 per cent decline in aerobic fitness per decade, which accounts for much of the loss of independence experienced by many older adults (Paterson et al., 1999). The decline in aerobic power $\dot{V}O_2max$ is likely a result of a reduced physical capacity, decline in physiological systems, and increased morbidity. The decline in aerobic power with age is well documented, but the estimated rate of decline varies widely among individuals and is contingent upon the influence of physiological factors (Table 9.1). Recent publication of longitudinal data addressing age-associated cardiorespiratory function reports that an annual $\dot{V}O_2max$ decline in men of –0.43 mlAkg^{-1}Amin^{-1} per year (14.7% per decade) and –0.19 mlAkg^{-1}Amin^{-1}per year (7.0% per decade) in older women (Stathokostas et al., 2004). There is also a parallel decline for ventilatory threshold (T_{VE}); however, the rate of decline is less than that observed for $\dot{V}O_2max$, –0.14 (2.5% per decade) for older men and –0.11 (1.0% per decade) for older women (Stathokostas et al., 2004). Therefore, the ability of older adults to perform submaximal aerobic work may be reduced at a slower rate than that observed with $\dot{V}O_2max$. As a result of its slower decline, the T_{VE} is reached at a higher percentage of $\dot{V}O_2max$ in older adults compared to young adults. Therefore, older adults who chose to exercise at their ventilatory threshold (moderate-vigorous intensity), for periods of 30 minutes or longer will slow and/or even reverse age-associated functional deterioration (American College of Sports Medicine, 1998). Such training stimulus is needed in order for older adults to extend and/or preserve years of active/independent life expectancy (Cunningham et al., 1987).

Table 9.1 ***Age-related Cardiorespiratory Limitations to Exercise***

Central Factors	*Peripheral Factors*
cardiac output	PaO_2 due to pulmonary impairment
maximal stroke volume	redistribution of blood flow to active
contractile performance resulting in 8 end	muscle tissue
systolic and diastolic volume	muscle oxidative capacity
left vertical compliance	muscle mitochondrial number and density
heart rate maximum	
systemic blood pressure	

Muscular Fitness

The age-related loss of muscle strength is well documented (Young et al., 1985; Vandervoort and McComas 1986; Skelton et al., 1994). There is an estimated 40 per cent decrease in muscle cross-sectional area, (muscle atrophy), between the ages of 20–80 years (Lexall, 1993), and a concomitant reduction in the number of motor neurons affecting innovation to a variety of muscle groups (Galea, 1996). Although there is some variation in the degree of strength loss between muscle groups and in the rate of decline, most of the literature is in agreement that significant declines in muscle strength occurs between 70–79 years of age. The greatest declines occur in those muscles that are used less frequently, particularly in movements that demand high velocity contraction during muscle shortening (concentric) rather than lengthening (eccentric) (Vandervoort, 2002). Nevertheless, age-related remodelling of the neuromuscular system does not have to be an inevitable consequence of ageing, and research suggests that much of the age-related strength loss is due to lifestyle factors (inactivity, malnutrition). Individuals who continue to regularly use certain muscles, either through exercise or their occupation, are able to slow the age-related decline in strength. Even more encouraging is the plethora of evidence that supports the long-term trainability of older muscle (McCartney et al., 1995), even in those considered frail and living with significant comorbidity (Fiatarone et al., 1994).

If we are to be successful in promoting the benefits of strength training in the geriatric population, we have to be able to demonstrate that an increase in strength will result in an improvement in daily independence and functional performance. It has been suggested that a healthy 80-year old woman is at or very close to, the threshold level of quadriceps strength required to rise from a common armless chair, whereas the same movement would demand only a 50 per cent effort in a young sedentary female (Young et al., 1986). Even a 10–20 per cent increase in strength would be enough to postpone this 80-year old woman from dropping below this critical threshold. It is important to recognize that even a minor gain in strength may result in significant improvements in things like independent ambulation and/or performance of self-care activities. It is encouraging to note that significant correlations have been found between leg strength and functional tasks, such as walking speed, rising up from a chair, and climbing stairs (Bassey et al., 1992). These observations certainly support the use of high-intensity resistance training as a method to improve both strength and functional performance in the geriatric population.

Although it appears that there are certain unavoidable changes that occur within the cardiorespiratory and neuromuscular systems, it is possible to delay or attenuate the losses through exercise. Since independent performance of many activities of daily living, is dependent upon cardiorespiratory and muscular fitness, it is important to minimize the age-related loss as much as possible. Older adults continue to retain their ability to adapt to training, regardless of past exercise history. This suggests that it may never be too late for older adults to incorporate daily exercise into their lifestyle; exercise is of universal importance.

Exercise for Frail Older Adults

Frail older adults, who cannot attend a formal aerobic exercise programme can simply march in-place, walk from room-to-room in their home or back-and-forth in the hallway of their apartment building. Starting with five minutes of continuous activity, increasing the frequency (number of times per week), intensity (moderate to vigorous) and duration will allow the frail older adult to preserve their remaining functional abilities, delaying the need for additional care and early nursing home admission. Recent evidence suggests that home exercise programmes are an effective means of reducing functional decline in frail older adults (Gill et al., 2002; Tudor-Locke et al., 2000). Bed rest, because of injury and/or illness, can severely decondition an older adult, making recovery and rehabilitation a long and slow process. However, those with stable health conditions can perform aerobic activities throughout the recovery period by using arm ergometers or resistive pulleys.

Continuous versus Accumulated Activity

Current health promotion recommendations suggest that one can accumulate 30, 60 or 90 minutes of activity, and this may be accomplished through shorter bouts or 'bursts' of activity completed throughout the course of the day. Epidemiological data supports this theory for younger age groups; however, this may not hold true for older adults whose cardiorespiratory system takes almost 3x longer to reach a steady aerobic state (DeLorey et al., 2004). This blunted cardiorespiratory response has significant functional implications when used to perform normal daily physical activities that require short bursts of movement. An attenuated ability to reach an aerobic steady state will require the older adult to spend more time in an anaerobic state, thus short activity bouts, without sufficient warm-up, will likely cause early fatigue and reduction to daily activity levels. However, a proper warm-up that uses large muscle groups and continuous movement, such as walking, can help to improve oxygen kinetic speed in older adults, allowing them to maximize their aerobic exercise activities (Scheuermann et al., 2002). Without an appropriate warm-up older adults will find themselves trying to complete activities of daily living in an anaerobic state that will promote early fatigue and eventual limitations in activities of daily living. Therefore, older adults should perform continuous activity following a warm-up, in order to improve exercise tolerance and avoid early onset fatigue.

Fitness versus Physical Activity

Older adults can expect to live, on average, two to nine years in a state of dependent living (Katz et al., 1983). By 75 years of age simple activities (housework, gardening) become very fatiguing for the sedentary older adult, a result of poor aerobic fitness, and they will have to work near their maximal capacity just to complete simple daily activities (Figure 9.2). It has been estimated that the minimum $\dot{V}O_2max$ required to maintain an independent lifestyle is approximately 15–18 ml≅kg≅min^{-1} (Paterson et al., 1999). A vicious cycle begins whereby an older adult is less likely to perform fatigue-limiting activities, such as domestic housework and shopping, due to their limited aerobic capacity. The current evidence suggests that fitness is directly associated with dependence, and for each 1.0 ml≅kg≅min^{-1} decline in $\dot{V}O_2max$ there is a 14 per cent greater likelihood of becoming dependent in old age (Paterson et al., 2004). In essence the less fit become functionally dependent long before those who maintain and/or improve their aerobic fitness through regular exercise regardless of existing morbidity. Older adults who perform regular cardiorespiratory exercise can experience a 10 per cent or greater (3–4 ml≅kg≅min^{-1}) increase in $\dot{V}O_2max$. Improved fitness will reduce the likelihood of becoming dependent by 50 per cent (Paterson et al., 2004). Therefore, older individuals who either restore or preserve higher levels of aerobic fitness are likely to substantially reduce their chance of becoming dependent, and reduce their risk of cardiovascular disease. There is little evidence to support the notion that general leisure activities engaged in by older adults will reduce the odds of dependent living, but they may support the role of routine exercise, including walking, that may improve cardiorespiratory fitness.

Figure 9.2 ***Age-related Decline of VO_2 max and Ventilatory Capacity***

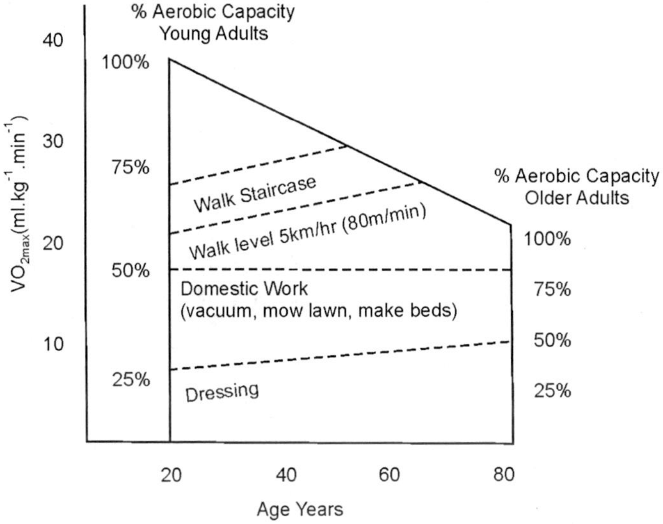

Health promotion activities primarily endorse physical activity as a means to avoid disease and all-cause mortality with little attention given to preventing the loss of functional independence associated with growing older. In fact, when interviewed about why they exercised, older adults consistently reported that exercise allowed them to remain functionally independent; some mentioned improved well-being while only a few cited exercise as a means of disease prevention (Estabrooks and Carron, 1999). A regular dose of aerobic exercise combined with strength training is likely the best prescription to postpone or prevent dependence in older adults and allow them to age gracefully (Dvorak et al., 2000).

Barriers to Physical Activity and Exercise

Persuading older adults to become physically active is a challenging task. Despite the known health benefits of regular exercise many older adults consider themselves too old or frail to participate in such activities (Schutzer and Graves, 2004). Exercise is rarely viewed as a necessary prescription medicine. In addition, older adults, due to a preponderance of health problems, encounter more barriers to physical activity and exercise participation. Regardless, of the excuse there exists a complex series of factors, which inhibit exercise participation (Brawley et al., 2003).

Regular exercise participation involves a complex and dynamic process involving an intricate series of behaviors, making identification of variables affecting exercise participation and adherence difficult. First, many older adults view the adoption of moderate exercise as time consuming (Chao et al., 2000). Also, older adults view exercise as a recreational pursuit instead of necessary medical therapy. Additionally, older adults often perceive exercise symptoms, such as sweating, laboured breathing, muscle soreness as negative. This problem is perpetuated by the fact that many allied health professionals do not have the training and knowledge to prescribe exercise. They do not even provide exercise guidelines or directions to the older adult patient. New initiatives that use the influence of health professionals to prescribe an *exercise pill* to patients have shown some promise in helping older adults to engage in regular exercise for their health.

Medical Consent?

Continuing with customary daily activities which may already include aerobic exercise, should not require medical advice unless underlying health problems exist. However, older adults who are new to exercise or are considering engaging in more challenging activities should speak with their family doctor before they begin. A doctor may order an exercise stress test to determine if any contraindications to exercise exist. An abnormal result may lead to further investigation but would not necessarily limit the older adult from exercise participation. An exercise threshold just below the intensity that elicited the abnormal event can be safely set. Not exercising often does more harm than good, regardless of cardiovascular risk (Manson et al., 2002). Similarly, chronic degenerative diseases such as arthritis may limit the results gathered from the exercise stress test, but should not prevent appropriate exercise prescription. Those with joint and balance problems may find water-based activities (swimming, aquabics) more suitable.

Physician-based Exercise

Recent investigations have helped to reduce older adults' fears and misconceptions about exercise by training primary care physicians to prescribe exercise to their elderly patients (Duncan et al., 2005; Petrella et al., 2003). Those patients who were prescribed exercise by their physician were able to experience a significant improvement in $\dot{V}O_2$max over those who were not counseled on exercise. Moreover, patients who received exercise prescriptions from the doctor were more confident to exercise (improved exercise self-efficacy), and were better suited for long-term exercise adherence than controls. Both studies commented that the provision of a strong support network (exercising peers) and access to community-exercise programmes had a strong influence on improving overall fitness and exercise adherence. However, one might question the qualifications and efficacy of local community exercise programmes in which patients are prescribed to attend.

International Curriculum Guidelines for Exercise Leaders of Older Adults

The International Curriculum Guidelines for Preparing Physical Activity Instructors for Older Adults is a consensus document that outlines major content areas, which experts recommend should be included in any entry-level training programme, with the goal of preparing physical activity instructors to work with older adults (Ecclestone and Jones, 2004). Endorsed by the World Health Organization, these guidelines can be applied to older adults across the continuum, from healthy older adults living independently in community settings, to functionally dependent older adults in long-term care. Advanced training is necessary for those interested in working with older adults with severe disabilities, co-morbidity and/or cognitive impairment in rehabilitation settings or managing and directing facilities. Such guidelines will help to provide consistency among instructor training programmes throughout the world.

There are many myths, fears and misunderstandings about aerobic exercise for older adults, but research in the last 25 years has clearly shown that taking part in aerobic activities reduces disease, increases fitness, and contributes to preserving function and independence. Improved fitness makes daily activities easier to do, allowing older adults to adopt an active lifestyle with improved vigour, and ultimately to experience a higher quality of life.

Recommendations

1. Systematic exercise improves health but most importantly it preserves/restores one's capacity to remain functionally independent, even in the oldest old.
2. A clear public health message is needed to promote the importance of fitness and the role of exercise, physical activity, and an active living lifestyle.

3. Misconceptions and barriers to exercise participation may be alleviated by prescriptions from health professionals.
4. National guidelines, and eventually standards of practice should be adopted to support effective and safe exercise interventions for all older adults, including the robust, restorable, and the frail.

References

American College of Sports Medicine. 1998. "Exercise and Physical Activity for Older Adults: Position Stand of the American College of Sports Medicine". *Medicine and Science in Sports and Exercise*, 30(6): 992–1008.

Bassey, E.J., E.F. Fiaterone, E.F. O'Neill, M. Kelly, W.J. Evans and L.A. Lipsitz. 1992. "Leg extensor power and functional performance in very old men and women". *Clinical Science*, 82: 321–327.

Blair, S.N., H.W. Kohl, R.S. Paffenbarger, D.G. Clark, K.H. Cooper and L.D. Gibbons. 1989. "Physical fitness and all-cause mortality: A prospective study in men and women". *Journal of the American Medical Association*, 262: 2392–2401.

Blair, S.N., H.W. Kohl, C.E. Bralow, R.S. Paffenbarger, L.W. Gibbons and C.A. Macera. 1995. "Changes in physical fitness and all-cause mortality: A prospective study of healthy and unhealthy men". *Journal of the American Medical Association*, 273: 1093–1098.

Brawley, L.R., W.J. Rejeski and A.C. King. 2003. "Promoting physical activity for older adults: The challenges for changing behavior". *American Journal of Preventative Medicine*, 25(3Sii): 172–183.

Brooks, G.A., N.F. Butte, W.M. Rand, J.P. Flatt and B. Caballero. 2005. "Chronicle of the Institute of Medicine physical activity recommendation: How a physical activity recommendation came to be among dietary recommendations". *American Journal of Clinical Nutrition*, 79 (Suppl.): 921S–930S.

Chao, D., C.G. Foy and D. Farmer. 2000. "Exercise adherence among older adults: Challenges and strategies". *Control Clinical Trials*, 21(Suppl.): 212S–217S.

Cunningham, D.A., P.A. Rechnitzer, J.H. Howard and A.P. Donner. 1987. "Exercise training of men at retirement: A clinical trail". *Journal of Gerontology*, 42: 17–23.

DeLorey, D.S., J.M. Kowalchuk and D.H. Paterson. 2004. "Effect of age on O_2 uptake kinetics and the adaptation of muscle deoxgenation at the onset of moderate-intensity cycling exercise". *Journal of Applied Physiology*, 97: 165–172.

Dvorak, R.V., A. Techernof, R.D. Starling, P.A. Ades, L. DiPietro and E.T. Poehlman. 2000. "Respiratory fitness, free-living physical activity, and cardiovascular disease risk in older individuals: A doubly labelled water study". *Journal of Clinical Endocrinology and Metabolism*, 85(3): 957–963.

Duncan, G.E., S.D. Anton, S.J. Sydeman, R.L. Newton, J.A. Corsica, P.E. During, T.U. Ketterson, A.D. Martin, M.C. Limacher and M.G. Perri. 2005. "Prescribing exercise at varied levels of intensity and frequency: A randomized controlled trial". *Archives of Internal Medicine*, 165: 2362–2369.

Ecclestone, N.A. and C.J. Jones. 2004. "International Curriculum Guidelines for Preparing Physical Activity Instructors for Older Adults". International Society for Aging and Physical Activity. Retrieved November 15, 2005, from http://www.isapa.org/guidelines/index.cfm

Estabrooks, P.A. and A.V. Carron. 1999. "The effects of group cohesion on older adult exercisers: From theory to practice". *Journal Behavioural Medicine*, 22(6): 575–588.

Fiatarone, M.A., E.C. Marks, N.D. Ryan, C.N. Meredith, L.A. Lipsitz and W.J. Evans. 1990. "High intensity strength training in nonagenarians: Effects on skeletal muscle". *Journal of the American Medical Association*, 263: 3029–3034.

Franco, O.H., C. de Laet, A. Peeters, J. Jonker, J. Mackenbach and W. Nusselder. 2005. "Effects of physical activity on life expectancy with cardiovascular disease". *Archives of Internal Medicine*, 165: 2355–2360.

Galea, V. 1996. "Changes in motor unit estimates with aging". *Journal of Clinical Neurophysiology*, 13: 253–260.

Gill, T.M., D.I. Baker, M. Gottschalk, P.N. Peduzzi, H. Allore and A. Byers. 2002. "A program to prevent functional decline in physically frail, elderly persons who live at home". *New England Journal of Medicine*, 347(14): 1068–1074.

Goode, R.C., R. Mertins, H. Bell and J. Piccinini. 1999. "Voice, breathing sounds, just audible breathing the ventilatory threshold of exercise intensity". Proceedings from the 1999 ALCOA National Forum, pp. 73–76.

Katz, S., L.G. Branch, M.H. Branson and D.S. Greer. 1983. "Active life expectancy". *New England Journal of Medicine*, 309: 1218–1224.

Manson, J.E., P. Greenland, A.Z. LaCroix, M.L. Stefanick, C.P. Mouton, A. Oberman, M.G. Perri, D.S. Sheps, M.B. Pettinger and D.S. Sisovick. 2002. "Walking compared with vigorous exercise for the prevention of cardiovascular events in women". *New England Journal of Medicine*, 347(10): 716–725.

McCartney, N., A.L. Hicks, J. Martin and C.E. Webber. 1995. "Long-term resistance training in the elderly: Effects of dynamic strength, exercise capacity, muscle and bone". *Journal of Gerontology: Biological Sciences*, 50A: B97–B104.

Morey, M.C., C.F. Pieper and J. Cornoni-Huntley. 1998. "Physical fitness and functional limitations in community-dwelling older adults". *Medicine and Science in Sports and Exercise*, 30: 715–723.

Morris, J.N., M.G. Everitt, R. Pollard, S.P.W. Chave and A.M. Semmence. 1980. "Vigorous exercise in leisure-time: Protection against coronary heart disease". *Lancet*, 8: 1207–1210.

Murtagh, E.M., B.A. Colin, A.G. Boreham and M.H. Murphy. 2002. "Speed of exercise intensity of recreational walkers". *Preventive Medicine*, 35: 397–400.

Myers, J., M. Prakash, V. Froelicher, Dat Do, S. Partington and J.E. Atwood. 2002. "Exercise capacity and mortality among men referred for exercise testing". *New England Journal of Medicine*, 346(11): 793–801.

Paterson, D.H., D.A. Cunningham, J.J. Koval and C.M. St. Croix. 1999. "Aerobic fitness in a population of independently living men and women aged 55 to 86". *Medicine and Science in Sports and Exercise*, 31(12): 1813–1820.

Paterson, D.H., D. Govindesamy, M. Vidmar, D.A. Cunningham and J.J. Koval. 2004. "Longitudinal study of determinants of dependence in an elderly population". *Journal of the American Geriatrics Association*, 52: 1632–1638.

Petrella, R.J., J.J. Koval, D.A. Cunningham and D.H. Paterson. 2003. "Can primary care doctors prescribe exercise to improve fitness? The Step Test Exercise Prescription (STEP) project". *American Journal of Preventative Medicine*, 24(4): 316–322.

Scheuermann, B.W., C. Bell, D.H. Paterson, T.J. Barstow and J.M. Kowalchuk. 2002. "Oxygen uptake kinetics for moderate exercise are speeded in older humans by prior heavy exercise". *Journal of Applied Physiology*, 92: 609–616.

Schutzer, K.A. and B.S. Graves. 2004. "Barriers and motivations to exercise in older adults". *Preventative Medicine*, 39: 1056–1061.

Skelton, D.A., C.A. Greig, J.M. Davis and A. Young. 1994. "Strength, power and related functional ability of healthy people aged 65–89 years". *Age and Ageing*, 23: 317–377.

Tudor-Locke, C., A.M. Myers, C.S. Jacob, G. Jones, D.A. Lazowski and N.A. Ecclestone. 2000. "Development and formative evaluation of the Centre for Activity and Ageing's Home Support Exercise Program for frail older adults". *Journal of Aging and Physical Activity*, 8: 59–75.

Vandervoort, A.A. and A.J. McComas. 1986. "Contractile changes in opposing muscles of the human ankle joint with aging". *Journal of Applied Physiology*, 61: 361–367.

Vandervoort, A.A. 2002. "Aging of the human neuromuscular system". *Muscle and Nerve*, 25: 17–25.

Wang, B.W.E., D.R. Ramey, J.D. Schettler, H.B. Hubert and J.F. Fries. 2002. "Postponed development of disability in elderly runners: A 13-year longitudinal study". *Archives of Internal Medicine*, 162: 2285–2294.

Young, A.M., M. Stokes and M. Crowe. 1986. "Exercise physiology in the geriatric practice". *Acta Medica Scandinavia*, 711: 227–232.

10 Nutrition for Healthy Ageing

Seema Puri

The increasing number of aged people worldwide has rendered human ageing and longevity a major area of scientific research. As we all know, ageing is an inevitable, irreversible and progressive phenomenon and is the last phase of the human life cycle. It is characterized by functional decline ultimately leading to death. Advancing age is accompanied by progressive physiological changes in the function of most organs. As people age, there also tends to be a concomitant increase in the presence and number of chronic conditions such as hypertension, cardiovascular disease, osteoporosis, diabetes and dementia among others. These further compromise the quality of life in old age.

In order to live longer and healthier lives, it would therefore not only be necessary to delay the process of physiological ageing but also to prevent/delay the imposition of pathological ageing (in the form of chronic degenerative diseases) on an individual. Another important issue related to longevity is ensuring a good quality of life among the oldest old. While lower morbidity would reduce mortality, compression of morbidity into a lesser time frame would ensure a life with minimum disability and frailty, a life of dignity and independence.

Nutrition is coming to the fore as a major modifiable determinant of chronic diseases and age-related decline. Scientific evidence increasingly supports the view that alterations in the diet have strong effects, both positive and negative, on health throughout life. Most importantly, dietary adjustments may not only influence present health but may determine whether or not an individual will develop diseases like cancer, cardiovascular disease and diabetes much later in life.

Physiological Ageing

Ageing is associated with a decline in many body functions, an accompanying change in structure, loss of lean mass and a relative increase in fat mass over time. While in previous years these changes were considered to be intrinsically due to ageing, research over the past several decades has increasingly ascribed them to age-related disuse, inactivity and degenerative diseases. These physiological and structural changes influence food and nutrient intakes, food preferences and the diet patterns of older persons. The nutritional requirements also undergo considerable change with advancing age.

(a) *Changes in body composition:* Some of the most dramatic changes seen with age are in body composition. Lean body mass declines over the adult age span and the decline accelerates beyond 80 years. Sarcopenia, a deficiency of flesh or muscle, strongly influences muscle strength, gait and balance, contributing to the increased risk of falls and frailty in older persons (Dutta, 1997). Sarcopenia develops even in healthy, successfully ageing adults and does not depend on the onset of disease. Its multifactorial etiology includes biological changes of ageing, disuse atrophy secondary to declining physical activities and in some cases, protein or energy undernutrition or catabolic disease processes such as congestive heart failure, rheumatoid arthritis, hyperthyroidism, Parkinson's disease, and chronic infection.

Fat mass increases two-fold between 20 and 60 years of age, followed by progressive decline. High fat mass is a risk factor for many diseases affecting older persons, including coronary heart disease, high blood pressure, diabetes, gallstones, osteoarthritis, and cancers of the breast and prostate. Increased obesity, especially distributed in the abdominal area, is associated with insulin resistance, which in turn causes diabetes and may also play a role in hypertension and hyperlipidaemia.

A positive energy balance, i.e., energy intakes exceeding energy expenditure, can explain the increase in body fat mass through middle age. Conversely, negative energy balance is the primary cause of loss of body fat in old age. Since protein balance is closely linked to energy balance, this negative energy balance may also be the cause of loss of body protein in old age even when a protein-adequate diet is consumed.

Consequent to these changes in body composition, alterations in body weight are also observed. Body weight increases during adult life until 50–59 years, after which it is seen to decline, particularly in the next two decades. Further, a reduction in lean body mass and decline in body weight leads to a decrease in basal metabolic rate, as age increases. Coupled with a decrease in physical activity, it leads to a reduction in energy requirements and consequently in the quantum of the food to be eaten.

(b) *Changes in bone health:* Ageing is typically associated with a loss of bone and total body calcium. Women at all ages have lower total bone mass or total body calcium than men. Over a lifetime, women lose about 40 per cent of their skeletal calcium, approximately one half in the first five years after menopause and the remainder at a slower rate thereafter. During the five years following menopause, calcium supplementation does not prevent bone mineral loss, whereas later postmenopausal women benefit significantly from it. As high dietary levels of sodium and protein increase urinary calcium excretion and thus more bone resorption, consumption of liberal amounts of processed foods, which are typically high in both sodium and protein, may contribute to the difficulty of maintaining bone mass in older persons.

The implications of poor bone health in older persons are related to an increased fracture risk and the effect on their functional ability and quality of life. In most cases hip fractures result from an injurious fall in persons with osteopenia. Prevention of hip fracture thus requires attention to both fall-related risk factors and bone density. Nutritional factors associated with traumatic hip fractures include protein-calorie malnutrition, alcohol abuse, osteomalaecia, low BMI, low muscle mass and strength, low levels of body fat, and low amounts of soft-tissue padding over the greater trochanteric region (WHO, 2002).

(c) *Immune function:* Considerable evidence indicates that ageing is associated with altered regulation of the immune system, which contributes to the increased incidence of infectious, inflammatory and neoplastic diseases observed in older persons, and to their prolonged post-illness recovery periods. The illness patterns in the elderly reflect both a deterioration of immune function and increased incidence of upper respiratory infections, tuberculosis and cancer. Several investigators have suggested that the nutritional status of older persons may be less than optimal, thereby contributing to immunological changes. Many macro- and micronutrients such as protein, zinc and vitamins E, C, and B_6, have been shown to play a regulatory role in immune system maintenance.

(d) *Neurological and cognitive function:* The age-associated increase in mental impairment leading to dementia is probably the most serious threat to ageing populations. Mental impairment and dementia as a result of chronic degenerative brain disease have a particularly severe impact on autonomy and independence. Depression, fairly common in older adults, may be associated with failing health, loss of independence, social isolation, financial concerns, grief over death of near and dear ones etc. Depression can affect appetite, dietary intake, digestion, weight status, fatigue and the overall sense of well-being (Harris, 2004).

It is generally accepted that dementating illnesses and depression have a strong genetic background. Nevertheless, since the genetic susceptibility to a certain disease is strongly influenced by environmental factors, nutrients can have either a disease-accelerating or a protective effect. For example, independently of genetic predisposition, certain nutrients or toxic substances can directly affect brain development (alcohol, folic-acid deficiency) or brain function (alcohol, vitamin B_1 and B_{12} deficiencies). Also, nutrition can have an impact on brain function by impairing energy supply; affecting neurotransmitter synthesis and intermediary metabolism; enhancing, or protecting from, oxidative stress; and influencing cytokines. Mental symptoms such as cognitive impairment, emotional irritability or other neurological signs are well known in cases where there are vitamin deficiencies.

Several studies suggest that mild or sub-clinical vitamin deficiency plays a role in the pathogenesis of declining neurocognitive function with age. Healthy older adults with low blood levels of some vitamins—particularly folate, vitamin B_{12}, vitamin C and riboflavin—have been found to score poorly on tests of memory and non-verbal abstract thinking. Significant correlations have also been reported between poor indices of thiamine, riboflavin and iron nutriture and impaired cognitive performance. The inverse correlation between plasma homocysteine levels and carotid artery stenosis suggests that low B-vitamin status may be related to the risk of cerebrovascular disease, with its associated changes in cognitive function. High-dose vitamin E supplementation appears to delay the progression of Alzheimer's disease, although scientists have not yet identified why vitamin E, other antioxidants, and other food factors, may have an effect on the illness (WHO, 2002).

(e) *Alterations in taste sensitivity:* Elderly people who have enjoyed food throughout their lives may experience a real decline in the quality of life because of changes in sensitivity to taste and smell. Both senses become less discriminating in old age, causing food to taste and smell less appetizing than it did previously. Approximately 25 per cent of adults over 65 years of age have a reduced ability to detect one or more of the four basic tastes (sweet, sour, salty and bitter) due to a reduction in the number and function of the taste buds in the tongue. Sensitivity to bitter and sour taste lasts longer than to sweet or salty taste. Furthermore, the olfactory bulbs in the brain begin to shrivel which reduces the ability to smell. This makes food taste even blander.

The loss of taste and smell sensitivity has an unfortunate side effect. Because food does not taste as good, older people suffer from loss of appetite, eat less and open the door to malnutrition. They oversalt their food thereby increasing their chances of developing hypertension. The decrease in sensitively to taste and smell robs the elderly of life's simple pleasures, e.g., smell of flowers, enjoyment of a good meal etc. (Puri, 2001).

(f) *Difficulty in feeding:* As one grows older there is a decline in neuromuscular coordination and proper handling of food, holding of utensils, and even self-feeding may become difficult. The elderly may therefore simplify their cooking procedures and eating patterns. Lack of mobility may also influence the ability to procure and prepare meals leading to significant dietary changes and nutritional inadequacies.

In addition, loss of teeth, faulty dentures or even no dentures significantly alters the type of food eaten. The diet may be soft and mushy, with raw vegetable and fruits and other hard to chew foods avoided. Consequently, a deficiency of vitamins and minerals as well as fibre may arise.

(g) *Gastrointestinal tract changes:* After the age of 50, there is a reduction in salivary secretion and a reduction in ptyalin content. Hence, the digestion of complex carbohydrates is affected. Gastric pepsin secretion as well as acid secretion decreases, and gastric volume is reduced. Delayed emptying of the stomach is seen in the elderly. Intestinal motility is reduced due to atrophy of gastrointestinal tract musculature. Such changes in the alimentary tract lead to altered food intake and avoidance of many foods. Constipation and flatulence are common complaints among the elderly (Puri, 2001).

Pathological Ageing

Coupled with age-related physiological decline is the imposition of chronic degenerative diseases in old age, e.g., hypertension, cardiovascular disorders, diabetes and cancers. In fact, multiple morbidities are very commonly found in this age group. Furthermore, "clustering" of these diseases towards the terminal part of life is a common phenomenon.

(a) *Coronary heart disease and stroke:* Coronary heart disease and stroke have become the major causes of death and disability among both ageing women and men. Proper food intake, particularly reduced intake of total and saturated fat and increased intake of plant food, is a cornerstone in preventing and managing coronary risk factors, notably lipoprotein disorders, and in protecting against arterial damage, whether by oxidation or other means. A number of food factors may afford cardio-protection through various pathways such as endothelial function, platelet aggregation, blood pressure, homocysteinaemia and cardiac membrane electrical stability. These include micronutrients such as folate and vitamins B_6 and B_{12}, which lower homocysteine levels; *n*–3 fatty acids, which decrease platelet aggregation; and vitamins C and E and phytochemicals, which are antioxidants for lipoprotein, deoxyribonucleic acid (DNA) and all cell membrane phospholipids (WHO, 2002).

Animal fat, saturated fatty acids and total fat intakes have been positively related to the risk of cerebral infarct in some studies. Folate and vitamin B6 have an important role in stroke prevention. Many observers consider that plant-derived foods may protect against stroke, probably for several reasons including by the lowering of blood pressure. Vitamin E has been associated with a reduced risk of ischaemic stroke but an increased risk of haemorrhaegic stroke. Alcohol is known to increase stroke risk in a linear fashion.

(b) *Cancer:* Analysis of the risk factors involved in the development of major cancers shows that a few such factors dominate—tobacco, diet, alcohol, infections and hormones; fortunately, all lend themselves to preventive action.

A high intake of total fat increases the risk of some types of cancer—cancer of the breast, the colon, the prostate, rectum and ovaries. Other dietary factors, including intake of alcohol; charred, smoked, and salt- and nitrate-cured foods; and naturally occurring contaminants such as aflatoxins and N-nitroso compounds also pose a potential risk for cancer. Food-intake patterns emphasizing unrefined foods high in dietary fibre are associated with low rates of certain cancers, especially of the breast and colon. Fruits and green and yellow vegetables, which are important sources of antioxidant vitamins, chemo-preventive phytochemicals, and dietary fibre are also associated with reduced risk of several forms of cancer. For example, vitamin C appears to have a protective effect against oesophageal, stomach, cervical, breast and lung cancers.

(c) *Osteoporosis and bone fractures:* Osteoporosis and associated bone fractures often result in enormous medical expense, and are one of the major causes of disability and death the world over. The number of osteoporotic fractures increases exponentially with age. In India, unlike the senile osteoporotic fractures of the West, the high fluoride, low calcium dietaries and post-menopausal loss of bone density may be contributing factors for developing osteoporosis (Puri, 2001).

Women are more prone to osteoporosis because their bone loss accelerates after menopause. While estrogen deficiency is the primary cause, especially in elderly women, factors such as diet, physical activity and smoking are closely associated with osteoporosis. Lifestyle modifications, particularly increased calcium intake and physical activity, could over time have an important preventive impact on fracture rates.

There is substantial evidence that calcium and vitamin D protect against osteoporosis. High calcium intake during the early years contributes to greater peak bone mass. During the later years, calcium, together with vitamin D, prevents negative calcium balance and reduces the rate of bone loss. In addition to calcium, other minerals including boron, copper, magnesium, manganese and zinc appear to contribute to the maintenance of bone density with age. Sodium adversely affects calcium balance through the promotion of urinary calcium loss (Goulding et al., 1986). There is increasing evidence that phytoestrogens from soy and some other plant sources may account for better bone health in patients than might otherwise be expected given their calcium intake (Dalais et al., 1998). Other nutrients such as vitamin K and essential fatty acids also contribute to bone health. Although they are not as well established, dietary risk factors for osteoporosis include excessive consumption of caffeine, protein and alcohol (Heaney, 1987). Thus, as in other chronic noncommunicable diseases, an overall food pattern is likely to be more important for bone health among older persons than any single food factor taken alone.

(d) *Other chronic conditions:* A growing body of evidence suggests that preventive nutrition strategies may also play a significant role in other chronic conditions which, while not necessarily directly associated with risk of fatality, do affect independence, quality of life and health care expenditure. For example, studies have demonstrated that supplementation with antioxidant vitamins, vitamin B_6, zinc and/or multivitamin/mineral formulations can enhance immune response in older persons, and thus reduce risk and duration of infectious disease episodes. Body fat and its abdominal distribution are consistently related to the prevalence of Type II diabetes whereas diet, weight loss and exercise can normalize blood sugar levels in most patients and delay the onset of diabetic complications. Obesity exacerbates conditions such as rheumatoid arthritis, and osteoarthritis, which are highly prevalent among older persons. Evidence also suggests an important relationship between the incidence of age-related cataract and nutritional status, particularly where the antioxidant vitamins C and E are concerned. Recently, epidemiological studies have indicated an inverse association between generous intakes of dietary carotenoids (especially lutein and zeaxanthin from foods such as corn and eggs) and vitamins C and E, and the incidence of age-related macular degeneration. Age-related mascular degeneration is the leading cause of irreversible blindness among older adults (Seddon et al., 1994).

(e) *Drug-nutrient interactions*: In addition to the disease, many medications administered often have strong repercussions on the health and nutriture of the ageing persons. Many prescription drugs are known to precipitate nutrient deficiencies by causing a reduction in nutrient intake, a decrease in nutrient availability, an inhibition of nutrient transport across intestines, a metabolic antagonism, an increase in nutrient catabolism and an increase in nutrient losses. The aged, particularly those with chronic debilitating disorders are at greater risk. Alcoholism also influences food and nutrient intakes and may lead to a deficiency of several vitamins and minerals.

The Nutrition Transition

It is a well established fact that the health of an individual, and the population in general, is the result of interactions between genetics and a number of environmental factors; nutrition being of major importance. Our genetic profile has not changed over the past 10,000 years, whereas major changes have taken place in our food supply and in energy expenditure and physical activity. Concomitantly, a sharp rise in the prevalence of noncommunicable diseases (NCDs) like diabetes, hypertension, cardiovascular diseases and cancers has been observed.

What is apparent at the global level is that great changes have swept the entire world since the second half of the 20th century, inducing major modifications in diet, first in industrial regions and more recently in developing countries. The nutrition transition itself is marked by a shift from relatively monotonous diets based on indigenous staple grains or starchy roots, locally grown legumes, other vegetables and fruits, and (except for prosperous subpopulations) limited foods of animal origin, towards more varied diets that include more preprocessed food, more foods of animal origin, more sugar and fat, especially in processed drinks and foods, and often more alcohol. Shifts in the dietary structures include a greater role for fat and added sugars in foods, greater saturated fat intake (mostly from animal sources), reduced intake of complex carbohydrates and dietary fibre and reduced fruit and vegetable intakes. These dietary changes are compounded by lifestyle changes that reflect reduced physical activity at work and during leisure. The most immediate result of the combination of such relatively energy-dense diets with physically inactive lives is a rapid increase in overweight and obesity.

The consequent epidemiological transition is from a predominance of endemic deficiency and infectious diseases, often caused or exacerbated by poor nutrition, to epidemic, chronic diseases. Diet-related chronic diseases include tooth decay, gastrointestinal disorders, obesity, adult-onset diabetes, hypertension, peripheral vascular disease and stroke, hyperlipidemia, angina and ischemic heart disease (IHD), and certain cancers. Most of these diseases also have nondietary causes; for example, the use of tobacco with lung cancer. There is also genetic predisposition to some of these diseases. The risk of this eventuating in overt clinical symptoms is increased by inappropriate environmental factors, including diet.

India also faces the repercussions of such a nutritional transition. Rapid urbanization and migration has brought about changes in traditional diet patterns and cooking methods, adversely affecting the health of the population. The increasing use of refined cereals, animal foods, sugar, salt and fat and the popularity of an ever increasing range of ready to eat, processed foods coupled with lower activity levels have also resulted in a concomitant increase in prevalence rates of obesity, heart disease, diabetes, hypertension etc. As expected, the urban population is affected more. Several studies have also established that the prevalence of such disorders is greater in certain ethnic groups like Punjabis and Gujaratis, Sikhs and Muslims. Diets of these communities are rich in dairy products, animal foods and fats particularly ghee (Gopinath et al., 1995). When people from these communities who settled in the West were studied, the prevalence rates of obesity, heart disease, diabetes, hypertension, etc. were higher, indicating that the adoption of the Western lifestyle and diet had a greater adverse effect.

A recent analysis of Census data by Gupta et al. (2005) revealed that CVD mortality rates were high in Andhra Pradesh, Tamil Nadu,

Punjab and Goa and low in Nagaland, Meghalaya, Sikkim and Himachal Pradesh. They found a significant positive correlation of CVD mortality with consumption of fat, milk and its products and sugar as well as with obesity and a significant negative correlation with green leafy vegetable intake. Moreover, fish-eating populations had lower blood cholesterol and LDL levels and higher HDL levels as compared to non fish-eating populations.

At the other extreme is the problem of inadequate nutrition which ranks as one of the major problems of old age. Varying estimates suggest that between 16 and 50 per cent of the elderly people do not have adequate nutrition and experience hunger everyday. Surprisingly, malnutrition is not confined to any one socio-economic group. The elderly who are at most nutritional risk are those who have disabilities that restrict their motility, are mentally confused, and are very old.

The NNMB (1990–91) report covering eight Indian states revealed that a sizable elderly population is suffering from chronic energy deficiency (CED). The problem of CED shows an increasing trend with age. Using a cut-off level of 18.5 for BMI as indicative for CED, it was observed that nearly 30 per cent of elderly men and women, 60–69 years of age, suffered from CED, while the percentage increased to above 38 per cent among the 70+ age group. Other Indian studies have reported that the incidence of CED is higher in females, in the rural elderly, and among the low and low-middle income groups of urban elderly.

Vitamins and minerals are the nutrients most likely to be lacking in an older person's diet; they are most adversely affected by multiple medications and drugs. Numerous investigations in various parts of India, have revealed that the diets of the elderly are deficient in energy, iron, vitamin A, and in certain B group vitamins like riboflavin and niacin. Few workers have also reported inadequacies of protein and calcium.

Iron deficiency anaemia in the elderly is multifactorial in etiology and may occur due to dietary iron inadequacy, impaired iron absorption, bleeding in the gastrointestinal tract due to consumption of anticoagulants, etc. High intakes of cereals, pulses, tea etc. which are rich in iron absorption inhibitors, and low consumption of vitamin C rich fruits and vegetables may also affect iron absorption adversely.

Nutrition for Healthy Ageing

The area, which has created utmost interest in ensuring healthy ageing, is the diet and nutrient intakes of individuals. Since antiquity, people have been searching for potions to preserve health and prolong life. Researchers have evaluated the influence of various diet patterns on ageing changes and length of life in both experimental animals and human epidemiological studies. Several concepts have emerged from these studies.

Energy: Studies on experimental animals have established that calorie restriction is an important measure for prolonging life span. Animals fed diets restricted in kilocalories yet adequate in protein, vitamins and minerals beginning at weaning and continuing through adulthood live 40 per cent longer than those given unlimited access to food. Chronic diseases like such as of heart and kidney also appear at a later age in the energy restricted animals. However, such studies have not been replicated in human subjects.

Although obesity in humans is associated with a shorter life expectancy, the extent of the effect is somewhat controversial. Some data have indicated that the mortality rate associated with being underweight is the same as the rate associated with moderate obesity, particularly in those older than 60 years of age. On one hand, epidemiological data strongly suggests that obesity is associated with several diet related non-communicable disorders like diabetes, coronary heart disease (CHD) and malignancies and is a health risk for the elderly leading to early mortality. On the other hand, loss of weight and frailty also has negative connotations on the quality of life in old age.

Energy requirements generally decrease with age because of changes in body composition, including a decrease in basal metabolic rate (BMR) and a reduction in physical activity. WHO (2002) has recommended that since low levels of physical activity and unchanged levels of energy absorption typically accompany older age, lower energy intakes are required to prevent obesity. The energy requirements of old age appear to be 1.4 to 1.8 multiples of the BMR to maintain body weight at different levels of physical activity. Levels of physical activity that result in energy requirements in the higher end of the range are desirable for reducing morbidity and mortality. Translated into quantitative estimates, an intake of less than 1,500 kcals daily may give rise to health problems in the elderly.

Proteins: Protein intake, in addition to energy intake influences both rate of growth and survival. In experimental animals, diets high in energy and protein result in rapid growth, large body size and weight, and early onset of degenerative disease. The suggestion that rapid growth and increased body weight accelerate both physiological and pathological ageing has serious implications for humans in light of current growth patterns. Today's children are taller, heavier, and reach puberty at earlier ages than did previous generations.

Table 10.1 ***Recommended Daily Nutrient Intakes (WHO, 2002)***

Energy: 1.4–1.8 multiples of BMR to maintain body weight at different levels of physical activity.		
Protein: 0.9–1.1 g/kg		
Fat: 30 per cent in sedentary older persons and 35 per cent for active older persons. Saturated fats should not exceed 8 en per cent.		
Riboflavin: 1.3 mg for men and for 1.1 mg for women.		
Folate: 400 Fg		
Vitamin B_{12}: 2.5 Fg		
Vitamin C: 60–100 mg		
Vitamin A: 600–700 Fg retinol equivalents		
*Vitamin D:*10–15 Fg		
*Vitamin E:*100–400 IU		
Vitamin K: 60–90 Fg		
Calcium: 800–1200 mg (in the presence of adequate vitamin D nutrition)		
*Iron:*10 mg assuming there are no excessive iron losses		
Selenium: 50–70 Fg		
Zinc: High Zn availability (50+%)	Men 4.2 mg	Women 3.0 mg
Moderate Zn availability (30%)	Men 7.0 mg	Women 4.9 mg
Low Zn availability (15%)	Men 14.0 mg	Women 9.8 mg

As people age and experience a loss of skeletal tissue mass, stores of protein in skeletal muscle may be inadequate to meet the body's needs, making dietary protein intake more important. Decreased food intake and sedentary lifestyles, along with reduced energy expenditure, become critical risk factors for malnutrition especially for insufficient intake of protein and micronutrients. WHO (2002) has therefore suggested that protein intakes of 0.9–1.1 g/kg body weight per day may be considered beneficial for healthy older persons. Lower intakes would, however, result in depletion of muscle mass and sarcopenia.

Carbohydrates: An abundant intake of carbohydrates is needed to protect protein from being used as a source of energy. Current dietary guidelines recommend that approximately 45–65 per cent of total daily calories should come from carbohydrates. Emphasis should be placed on increasing the intake of complex carbohydrate sources such as legumes, whole grains, vegetables and fruits to provide fibre, phytochemicals and essential minerals and vitamins.

Fat: One can relate a high fat intake, particularly saturated fat and cholesterol to increased morbidity and mortality risk. Besides obesity, a high fat consumption has been linked to CHD, stroke, certain cancers and even Alzheimer's disease. Hence reduction in fat and energy intake from a younger age will contribute immensely to healthy ageing.

Current dietary recommendations propose that 25–35 per cent of energy come from fats. According to WHO (2002), except where overweight or obesity are problems, there is no further health benefit gained from restricting the fat calories of older persons beyond 30 per cent for those who are sedentary, and 35 per cent for those who are active. Conversely, restricting fat to less than 20 per cent energy may affect the overall quality of the diet and negatively affect taste, satiety and intake. A high intake of fat (greater than 35% of calories) generally increases saturated fat intake and makes it more difficult to avoid consuming excess calories. A low intake of fats and oils (less than 20% of calories) increases the risk of inadequate intakes of vitamin E and of essential fatty acids and may contribute to unfavourable changes in high-density lipoprotein (HDL) blood cholesterol and triglycerides.

To meet the total fat recommendation of 20 to 35 per cent of calories, most dietary fats should come from sources of polyunsaturated and monounsaturated fatty acids The consumption of saturated fats should be minimized and should not exceed 8 per cent of total energy. While it is desirable to have a variety of fats in the diet, the emphasis should be on including monounsaturated and polyunsaturated fat sources in the diet. Sources of omega6 polyunsaturated fatty acids are liquid vegetable oils, including soybean oil, corn oil, and safflower oil. Plant sources of omega3 polyunsaturated fatty acids (linolenic acid) include soybean oil, canola oil, walnuts, and flaxseed. Eicosapentaenoic acid (EPA) and docosahexaenoic acid (DHA) are omega3 fatty acids that are contained in fish and shellfish. An optimal ratio of n–6 to n–3 fatty acids in the diet is believed to be 4:1. Plant sources that are rich in monounsaturated fatty acids include nuts and vegetable oils (e.g., canola, olive, high oleic safflower, and sunflower oils) that are liquid at room temperature.

A relatively new concern with respect to monounsaturated fatty acid consumption involves the concentration of trans-fatty acids in the diet. Elaidic acid (trans 18: 1n–9) is the principal trans-fatty acid in the diet. Trans-fatty acids are formed during the hydrogenation process, a process that converts vegetable oils to a semisolid state. Major sources of trans-fatty acids in the diet are baked products, processed foods, and margarines rich in hydrogenated fat or oil. There is evidence that increased trans-fatty acid consumption, in contrast with consumption of saturated fat, increases plasma concentrations of lipoprotein (a), an independent risk factor for CHD. They also have a deleterious effect on the plasma lipoprotein profile, elevating LDL-cholesterol and reducing HDL-cholesterol concentrations.

Minerals: Whereas overt mineral deficiencies are less common in healthy adults, sub-clinical nutrient deficiencies can develop. Poor mineral status in older persons may be attributed to inadequate intake, medications, and/or physiological changes that may affect the need of such nutrients.

Ageing is typically associated with a loss of bone and total body calcium, particularly in women. It has been suggested that in the presence of adequate vitamin D nutrition, calcium intakes in the range of 800–1,200 mg/day will result in both a beneficial effect on bone mineral density of the femur, neck and lumbar spine and a reduction in fracture rates. Potential benefits of high calcium intakes and various other health-related measures, e.g., reduced blood pressure and decreased risk of a colon cancer, may also be important, although data are insufficient to know for certain (WHO, 2002).

Iron requirements in women decrease after menopause, while those of men remain similar. Iron deficiency anaemia in old age is most likely to be related to blood loss from disease and medications, or to decreased absorption caused by medications, or to hypochlorhydria rather than to inadequate intakes.

Zinc status is especially important for older persons, who need to maintain their full immunocompetence. Intakes of zinc in older adults decrease in relation to a decrease in energy intake, and may be much below the required levels. Zinc deficiency is associated with impaired immune function, anorexia, loss of sense of taste, delayed wound healing and pressure ulcers. WHO (2002) has given the recommended intakes for dietary zinc for people over 65 years of age as 4.2 mg/day for men and 3.0 mg/day for women (high Zn availability (> 50%); 7.0 mg/day for men and 4.9 mg/day for women (moderate Zn availability (30%); 14.0 mg/day for men and 9.8 mg/day for women (low Zn availability (15%).

Sodium intakes are often associated with hypertension. Therefore it is prudent to limit dietary sodium to approximately 2–4g/day.

Vitamins: Several vitamins have been ascribed with significant anti ageing contributions. Antioxidant vitamins like vitamin E, C and carotenoids are known to display disease prevention properties for a number of diseases, ranging from cardiovascular disease and cancer to cataracts and macular degeneration. B group vitamins play an important role in maintaining cognitive ability and neuromuscular integrity as age advances.

It is thought that requirements of vitamin A are high in old age due to the possible role of provitamin carotenoids in disease prevention, e.g., cancer, and cardiovascular disease. However, three intervention studies have shown that high levels of b-carotene, taken alone, not only do not reduce the risk of cancer or cardiovascular disease; they in fact, increase the incidence of lung carcinoma in heavy smokers (Omenn et al., 1996; Hennekens et al., 1996; The Alpha-Tocopherol, Beta Carotene Cancer Prevention Study Group, 1994). Concern has also been expressed about a low margin of safety for preformed dietary vitamin A in older persons. Based on these considerations, it appears that 600–700 ug RE/day represents an adequate intake for older men and women.

Inadequate vitamin D intake can also lead to bone loss and increased risk of osteoporosis. There are many reasons for vitamin D malnutrition in older persons including low exposure to sunlight, poor skin response to sunlight, and decreased absorption or decreased hydroxylation of vitamin D. Studies have shown that 1.2 g of elemental calcium and 20 μg of vitamin D/day significantly reduced the risk of hip fractures in older women (Dawson-Hughes et al., 1991). According to US dietary recommendations, it appears that older persons need 10– 20 μg of vitamin D per day to ensure optimal bone health (Institute of Medicine, 1998).

Vitamin E is of interest as a protective antioxidant and membrane stabilizer. In addition, vitamin E intakes have been associated with a protective effect against cataract and cancer, Alzheimer's disease and cardiovascular disorders. However, further research is needed to determine the adequacy of current vitamin E recommendations for older persons. Most of the interest in vitamin E requirements has centred on the possible beneficial effects of pharmacological doses (60–400 IU/day) of the vitamin, which could not be achieved through an otherwise healthy diet.

High vitamin C in blood levels and/or intakes have been associated with a lower prevalence of senile cataract, higher high-density lipoprotein cholesterol concentrations and lower incidences of coronary artery disease (Frei, 1991). However, it appears that older persons do not have different vitamin C requirements from younger people and that an intake level of 60–100 mg/day is adequate (WHO, 2002).

Recently, a new marker of folate status – homocysteine levels – has come into widespread use. There is a great interest in the role of homocysteine as an atherogenic agent and the possibility that tissue folate deficiency could play an indirect role in atheromatous disease. Data from the Framingham Heart Study among older people demonstrated that serum homocysteine levels are correlated with dietary folate levels, and that serum homocysteine levels are high at dietary folate intakes of < 400 ug/day (Selhub et al., 1993). Large-scale intervention studies will be needed to show that administration of folate at this level or above will in fact diminish the risk of vascular disease.

Antioxidant nutrients: The role of antioxidant nutrients in preventing free radical damage has been well documented. Although a wide variety of antioxidants in foods contribute to disease prevention, the bulk of research has focussed on antioxidant nutrients like vitamin E, vitamin C, carotenoids and selenium. Green leafy vegetables and fruits are rich in these nutrients and hence most nutritionists emphasize a liberal intake of these foods in old age.

Besides its anti-ageing properties, vitamin E is known to afford protection against cancer ischemia, cataract, arthritis and certain neurological disorders. The protective effects of vitamin C extend to cancer, coronary artery disease, arthritis and ageing. Carotenoids, including B carotene, and selenium are associated with reduced risk of certain cancers. However, the general consensus is that liberal servings of fruits and vegetables are more beneficial than antioxidant pills or medication (Puri, 1999; Bagchi and Puri, 1998).

Phytochemicals: In addition to the recognized essential nutrients, there are many other food components—collectively known as phytochemicals—about which little is known but whose biological effects can lower the risk of major health problems such as cancer and heart disease. Their effects may be hormonal, anti-inflammatory, antimicrobial, anti-oxidant, anti-mutagenic or anti-angiogenic (Table 10.1). Phytochemicals, mostly phenolic acids and flavonoids, are found in garlic, onion, ginger, oats, soyabean, tea, certain herbs and spice and red wine. The presence of these antioxidants in such foods may be the reason for the anti-ageing properties associated with them.

Table 10.2 ***Phytochemicals in Foods***

Carotenoids in orange/green vegetables, red wine: Antimutagen antioxidant, anticarcinogen, immuno-enhancing
Flavonoids in green/yellow vegetables, soy: Antioxidant, anticarcinogen, estrogen, immuno-modulating
Polyphenolics in berries, oregano: Antioxidant, antibacterial
Catechins in green tea: Antimutagen, anticarcinogen
Isothiocyanates and indoles in cruciferous vegetables: Antimutagen
Allyl sulphides in garlic, onions: cholesterol lowering, anticarcinogen, antibacterial
Curcumin in turmeric: Anti-inflammator
Non digestible carbohydrates in vegetables and fruits: cholesterol lowering, stimulates growth of microbial flora

For this reason alone it is important to obtain essential nutrients through a food-based approach and not be dependent on vitamin and mineral supplements. It is clear that a wide variety of food cultures and cuisines can promote healthy ageing. The traditional nutrient based approach is limited in that it does not take into account the environmental, socio-economic and lifestyle context of eating. Nor does it adequately address the chemical complexity of foods and the interactions and synergies, whether between different foods or individual food components. On the other hand, the food based approach extends beyond nutrients and food groups; they include the way foods are produced (agriculture), prepared (cuisine), processed and developed (industry). They are therefore culture sensitive.

Diets for Healthy Ageing: Lessons from Diverse Cultures

In the 1960s Greeks, followed by the Japanese had the longest life expectancy in the world. The traditional Greek diet was associated with very low rates of coronary heart disease and cancers of the colon and breast. The intake of fish, legumes, cereals and alcohol in both countries was probably protective against coronary heart disease, whereas a high intake of salty foods/dishes contributed to increased risk of stroke and stomach cancer in Japan. Today the Japanese have the world's longest life expectancy, which has been attributed in part to their increased intake of fruit and fat and reduced intake of salty traditional dishes.

The adherence to the traditional Greek food pattern was found to be significantly associated with a lower overall mortality and longer survival. The traditional Greek food pattern, i.e., before 1960 consisted of a high intake of vegetables (particularly wild plants), fruits, nuts and cereals mostly in the form of sourdough bread rather than pasta; more olives and olive oil; less milk more cheese; more fish, less meat; moderate amounts of wine more so than other Mediterranean countries. What appears to be special about the Greek diet relative to the other Mediterranean diets is the content of bioprotective nutrients, specifically: 1) a more balanced intake of EFA from vegetable, animal and marine sources; a ratio of (n–6) to (n–3) fatty acids of ~ 2:1, instead of the 15:1 in Western and Northern Europe and 16.74: 1 in the United States; and 2) a diet rich in antioxidants, i.e., high amounts of vitamin C, vitamin E, ß–carotene, glutathione, resveratrol, selenium, phytoestrogens, folate, and other phytochemicals from green leafy vegetables; phenolic compounds from wine and olive oil; high intakes of tomatoes, onions, garlic and herbs, especially oregano, mint, rosemary, parsley and dill, which contain lycopene, allyl thiosulfinates, salicylates, carotenoids, indoles, monoterpenes, polyphenols, flavonoids and other phytochemicals used in cooking vegetables, meat and fish. Such a dietary pattern has been shown to be beneficial to health because it is associated with a reduced risk of cardiovascular disease and cancer (Simopoulos, 2001).

The relationship between diet and disease in Japan is more complex than we are led to believe. The Japanese diet is low in fat, high in carbohydrates, devoid of dairy foods and rich in soy foods, and for this reason the Japanese enjoy the longest life-span in the world, with much lower rates of heart disease, osteoporosis, breast and prostate cancer than many other countries. Close examination of the traditional Japanese diet proves that, although very different from Western diets, Japanese cuisine embodies all the principles of nourishing traditional foodways. It is rich in fat-soluble vitamins from seafood and organ meats and in minerals from fish broth, and contains plenty of lacto-fermented foods. Japanese preparation techniques eliminate most of the antinutrients in grains and legumes.

Elderly Okinawans of Japan have among the lowest mortality rates in the world from the multitude of chronic diseases of aging and as a result enjoy not only what may be the world's longest life expectancy but the world's longest health expectancy. Their good health in old age is mostly due to their lifestyle, diet, regular exercise, moderate alcohol use, avoidance of smoking, blood pressure control, and a stress-minimizing psychospiritual outlook. The Okinawan diet, rich in green tea, soy, fish, vegetables, fruit and whole grains, plays a large part, along with moderation. The Okinawans stay lean by eating a low-calorie, unrefined-complex carbohydrate diet, practicing calorie control in a cultural habit known as *hara hachi bu* (only eating until they are 80% full), and keeping physically active the natural way.

Besides the lower caloric intake, high vegetables/fruits consumption, higher intake of omega-3, mono-unsaturated fat, high fiber diet, high flavonoid intake play an important role in protection against stroke and cancer. Protective factors against fractures include high calcium intake by Okinawans in food and their natural drinking water, high vitamin D levels from exposure to sunlight, increased physical activity, especially at older ages, and a high intake of dietary flavonoids (estrogenic compounds from plant foods). Moreover, the large quantities of soy they consume (rich in phytoestrogens) protect the Okinawan women against menopause related complications such as hot flashes, hip fractures, or coronary heart disease.

Vegetarianism is the favoured way of life among most Indians and is increasingly being associated with a healthier lifestyle, lower morbidity and longer lifespan. Components of a healthy vegetarian diet include a variety of vegetables, fruits, whole grain cereals, legumes and nuts. The use of traditional herbs and spices further enhances the beneficial effects of such a diet. Numerous studies including the Seventh Day Adventists study (Beeson et al., 1989), show important and quantifiable benefits of the different components of vegetarian diets, namely the reduction of risk for many chronic diseases and the increase in longevity. Vegetarians have been reported to have lower body mass indices than nonvegetarians, as well as lower rates of death from ischemic heart disease. Vegetarians also show lower blood cholesterol levels, lower blood pressure, and lower rates of hypertension, type 2 diabetes, and prostate and colon cancer.

According to the American Dietetic Association, a vegetarian diet is defined as one that does not include meat, fish, or fowl. Components of a healthy vegetarian diet include a variety of vegetables, fruits, whole grain cereals, legumes and nuts. Vegetarian diets offer a number of nutritional benefits, including lower levels of total and saturated fat, cholesterol, and animal protein as well as higher levels of carbohydrates, fiber, magnesium, potassium, folate, and antioxidants such as vitamins C and E and phytochemicals. Vegetarians generally have a lower alcohol intake and a greater consumption of vegetables and fruits. While meat intake has been related to increased risk for a variety of chronic diseases, an abundant consumption of vegetables, fruits, cereals, nuts, and legumes all have been independently related with a lower risk for several chronic degenerative diseases, such as ischemic heart disease, diabetes, obesity, and many cancers.

It is now well-known that vegetables, fruit, grains, and nuts contain phytosterols and unsaturated fats that lower blood cholesterol concentrations. Some phytochemicals may affect plaque formation and may exert anti-inflammatory effects. These same foods contain dietary fiber, which also lowers blood cholesterol and may protect against colon cancer. In addition, the content of a number of antioxidant substances (e.g., tocopherols, ascorbate, carotenoids, saponins, and flavonoids) may reduce the risk of heart disease by preventing the oxidation of LDL cholesterol, and may also reduce the risk of cancer by preventing oxidative damage to nucleic acids and other cellular components. A variety of indoles and isothiocyanates that are present in or formed from cruciferous vegetables can help detoxify carcinogenic substances and may also inhibit conversion of procarcinogens to carcinogens (Sabate, 2003).

Foods and Longevity

Consumption of specific foods may also have a beneficial effect on health, e.g., whole grains, vegetables and fruits, fish, green tea, red wine, soy, nuts and seeds, garlic, turmeric and so on. Constituents like fibre and several phytochemicals in these foods bestow antioxidant, antimutagenic, anti-inflammatory, antibacterial and immuno-enhancing properties – all contributing to lowered disease risk and hence increased longevity. For example, high fruit and vegetable consumption has been consistently associated with protection against macular degeneration, visual loss, cataracts, respiratory disease, and breast, stomach and colorectal cancer.

Animal foods: While plant based foods are now associated with a lower chronic disease risk, animal foods are implicated in the causation of a variety of diseases including cardiovascular disease, renal disorders and cancer. Meat products contain no dietary fiber and often contain substantial quantities of cholesterol and saturated fats that raise LDL-cholesterol concentrations. Meats do not contain significant amounts of phytochemicals, although small quantities may be found as a consequence of the animals having eaten plants. Moreover, there is some evidence that the process of heating and cooking meats, particularly if there is any burning, may form compounds such as polycyclic aromatic hydrocarbons and heterocyclic amines that are carcinogenic. Consumption of meat has also been shown to increase faecal content of potentially carcinogenic *N*-nitroso compounds.

Whole grains: Long-term observational studies found reduced chronic disease risk associated with consumption of rye and of mixed whole grains (primarily wheat and oats, plus some corn and rice). Furthermore, the benefit was found with the phytochemical-rich cereal fiber found in the whole grain, when eaten as part of whole foods. It appears that phytochemicals that are located in the fiber matrix besides the fiber itself are responsible for the reduced risk. The glycemic load of the different grains could be a mediating factor. A diet with a high glycemic load has been shown to adversely affect serum lipids and has been implicated in CAD. One strategy for reducing dietary glycemic load is to replace refined grains with whole grains and legumes (Sabate, 2003).

Vegetables and fruits: Low fruit and vegetable intake is among the top 10 risk factors contributing to attributable mortality, according to evidence presented in World Health Report (2003). High fruit and vegetable consumption has been consistently associated with protection against mascular degeneration, visual loss, cataracts, respiratory disease, cardiovascular disorders, and breast, stomach, and colorectal cancer.

Eating a variety of vegetables and fruits clearly ensures an adequate intake of most micronutrients, dietary fibres and a host of essential non-nutrient substances. As well, increased fruit and vegetable consumption can help displace foods high in saturated fats, sugar or salt. A recent WHO/FAO expert consultation report on diet, nutrition and prevention of chronic diseases (1990) sets population nutrient goals and recommends an intake of a minimum of 400 g of fruits and vegetables per day for the prevention of chronic diseases such as heart diseases, cancer, diabetes and obesity. The report states that there is convincing evidence that fruits and vegetables decrease the risk for obesity, and evidence that they probably decrease the risk of diabetes and CVD.

Soyabean: Legumes play an important role in the traditional diets of many regions throughout the world. By contrast, in Western countries beans tend to play only a minor dietary role despite the fact that they are low in fat and are excellent sources of protein, dietary fiber, containing a variety of micronutrients and phytochemicals. Soybeans are unique among the legumes because they are a concentrated source of isoflavones. Isoflavones have weak estrogenic properties and the isoflavone genistein influences signal transduction. Soyfoods and isoflavones have received considerable attention for their potential role in preventing and treating cancer and osteoporosis, as well as reducing cholesterol levels in people with hypercholesterolemia and raise HDL levels.

Nuts: Perhaps one of the most unexpected and novel findings in nutritional epidemiology in the past decade has been that consumption of nuts like walnuts, almonds, pecans etc. seem to protect against ischemic heart disease (IHD). Frequency and quantity of nut consumption has been documented to be higher in vegetarian than in nonvegetarian populations. Nuts also constitute an important part of other plant-based diets, such as Mediterranean and Asian diets. Several studies have documented an association between nut consumption and a decreased risk of IHD. High nut consumption seems not only to decrease the lifetime risk of IHD but to postpone the development of the disease for several years (Sabate, 2003). The protective effect of nuts on IHD has been found in men and women and in the elderly. Importantly, nuts have similar associations in both vegetarians and nonvegetarians.

Herbs and spices: A number of traditional herbs and spices have been associated with longevity and the slowing down of age-related decline besides their disease preventing qualities. Garlic and turmeric are well known examples. Several phytochemicals in these foods bestow antioxidant, antimutagenic, anti-inflammatory, antibacterial and immuno-enhancing properties – all contributing to lowered disease risk and hence increased longevity. Brahmi, gingko biloba, ginseng and many others are also attributed with preventing age-related memory loss, vitality and health.

Dietary Guidelines for Older Persons

In light of these facts, WHO (2002) has outlined principles of food based dietary guidelines for older persons. These food based dietary guidelines for older persons emphasize the inclusion of healthy traditional vegetable and legume-based dishes where meat and nuts may be used only as condiments. The use of herbs and spices is encouraged, and the consumption of traditional dishes/foods that are heavily preserved/pickled in salt is to be limited.

The guidelines recommend a prudent selection of nutrient-dense foods such as fish, lean meat, liver, eggs, soy products (e.g., tofu and tempeh) and low-fat dairy products, yeast-based products, fruits and vegetables, herbs and spices, whole-grain cereals, nuts and seeds. Moreover, nuts, seeds, beans, olives and fatty fish would also cater to fat intake. Where refined fats are necessary for cooking, selection from a variety of liquid oils including those high in n–3 and n–6 fats (canola, soyabean and olive oil) is desirable. There is also a strong focus on increasing variety in foods to be eaten as well as preserving healthy traditional food related practices. As the dependence on easily available ready to eat foods is increasing, the rapidly growing processed food industry and fast food chains should make concerted efforts to shift from the ready availability of high fat convenience foods to meals which are low in animal fat and high in nutrients and phytochemicals.

Table 10.3 ***Food Based Dietary Guidelines For Older Persons (WHO, 2002)***

Emphasize healthy traditional vegetable- and legume-based dishes where meat and nuts are used as condiments.
Limit consumption of traditional dishes/foods that are heavily preserved/pickled in salt and encourage the use of herbs and spices.
Introduce healthy traditional foods or dishes from other cuisines (e.g., tofu in Europe and the tomato in Asia) to increase the variety of foods consumed.
Select nutrient-dense foods such as fish, lean meat, liver, eggs, soy products (e.g., tofu) and low-fat dairy products, yeast-based products (e.g., spreads), fruits and vegetables, herbs and spices, whole-grain cereals, nuts and seeds.
Consume fat from whole foods such as nuts, seeds, beans, olives and fatty fish. Where refined fats are necessary for cooking, select from a variety of liquid oils, including those high in n 0–3 and n–6 fats. Avoid fatty spreads.
Enjoy food and eating in the company of others. Avoid the regular use of celebratory foods (e.g., ice cream, cakes and pastries, mithai and confectioneries)
Encourage the processed food industry and fast-food chains to produce ready-made meals that are low in animal fats and high in nutrients and phytochemicals.
Eat several (5–6) small non-fatty meals. This pattern appears to be associated with greater food variety and lower body fat and blood glucose and lipid levels, especially if larger meals are eaten early in the day.
Transfer as much as possible of one's food culture, health knowledge and related skills to one's children, grandchildren and the wider community.

Conclusion

With a growing number of individuals surviving to enjoy their "renaissance years", there has been considerable interest in aspects related to longevity and maintaining quality of life in old age. The role of nutrition in preventing/delaying age-related decline, as well as in the imposition of chronic degenerative diseases in Indians needs to be further investigated in view of emerging data on their increased genetic susceptibility to such disorders.

Keeping in mind the wide diversity of foods consumed in different regions of India, the role of various dietary components in causation or prevention of chronic disease needs to be studied. In ancient literature, many foods have been assigned with antiageing and disease prevention properties, e.g., brahmi for memory enhancement and amla for disease prevention. Scientific trials need to undertaken to validate such claims. With our rich heritage of herbs and indigenous foods, efforts should be made to promote the use of such beneficial foods in the diets of the elderly. The example of "isabgol" is a classic one. It has been eaten by generations of older Indians for stomach complaints. Now the West is propagating that it has other benefits like improving lipid profile, weight reduction.

In India, the market today is flooded with innumerable nutritional supplements and foods boasting claims of anti-ageing, increased vitality, cholesterol lowering etc. In fact, antioxidants are being promoted as the new "mantra" for all kinds of old age problems. We need to research and authenticate such claims ourselves before conveying the right messages to the masses.

At the individual level, to ensure a good nutritional status among the elderly creating awareness assumes utmost importance. We must remember that good nutritional status in old age is the culmination of the food patterns and other lifestyle influences throughout life. Hence, awareness creation about healthy lifestyles should begin with the elderly of tomorrow, i.e., the young adults and the middle aged.

Programmes focusing on the special needs of the elderly need to be formulated and propagated. Self-help booklets, videocassettes etc. on health and nutrition related issues need to be developed and information disseminated. Food guides and diet manuals for the elderly need to be developed, keeping in mind regional differences. The role of traditional foods, use of herbs, and therapeutic foods need to be highlighted. Dietary messages may be spread through a variety of channels – TV, radio, handouts, self-help booklets, talks and discussions etc. The television has emerged as a favourite past time among the elderly and can be used as an effective medium for transmission of health and nutrition related messages. Spiritual and religious forums like "satsangs" can also be used to propagate such messages.

In India, unlike in the West, a majority of the elderly live at home and not in old age institutions. Even today, in spite of the changing socio-cultural environment, the family is the primary caregiver for the elderly. Hence, our emphasis must be on home based care or on evolving strategies to support families to take care of their elderly at home.

As our focus is on home based care of the older persons, we need to develop a support system for the informal and formal caregivers of the old. Solitary dwelling, disabled, or frail elderly people may require assistance in daily activities of food purchasing, cooking, serving or even feeding. "Granny-sitting" services like baby-sitting may become necessary in the not too distant future. Nutritional support workers may be able to provide such services. In fact, involving the "able" elderly in such activities may be beneficial for both – the able elderly develop a feeling of self-worth while the disabled elderly get the support and companionship they need. Facilities like home catering services, meals on wheels etc. may be encouraged for the elderly who are unable to prepare meals for themselves. Home visits by trained dietitians would also help identify elderly people who are at risk, allowing interventions to be planned in time.

As nutrition security is dependent on many social and economic factors, in our efforts to provide a better quality of life to the elderly it is imperative to strengthen their economic security. Provision of old age pension or other social security benefits may be a step in this direction. To promote the concept of productive ageing, programmes should be planned to utilize the expertise and skills of the elderly, and to maximise their contribution to the family and the community at large. In order to improve the nutritional status of the economically deprived elderly, the government along with the cooperation of NGOs may explore avenues like food coupons, feeding programmes or distribution of nutritional supplements for the older persons.

In conclusion, ensuring good nutrition for healthy ageing is a complex task encompassing not only food and nutrient intakes but also issues of economic and social relevance. Empowering the elderly economically, guaranteeing their place in the family, community and society are some ways of ensuring nutrition security. Coupled with these, maintaining functional competence and good health will go a long way in ensuring a good quality of life in old age.

References

Bagchi, K. and S. Puri. 1998. "Dietary Antioxidants in Health and Disease: A Review". *Eastern Mediterranean Journal of the World Health Organization*.

Beeson, W.L., P.K. Mills, R.L. Phillips, M. Andress and G.E. Fraser. 1989. "Chronic Disease among Seventh-Day Adventists, A Low Risk Group". *Cancer*, 64: 570–581.

Dalais, F. et al. 1998. "Effects of dietary phytoestrogens in postmenopausal women". *Climacteric*, 1: 124–129.

Dawson-Hughes, B. et al. 1991. "Effect of vitamin D supplementation on wintertime overall bone loss in healthy postmenopausal women". *Annals of Internal Medicine*, 115: 505–512.

Dutta, C. 1997. "Significance of sarcopenia in the elderly". *J Nutr*, 127 (Suppl.): 992.

Frei, B. 1991. "Ascorbic acid protects lipids in human plasma and low-density lipoprotein against oxidative damage". *Am J Clin Nutr*, 54: S1113–S1118.

Gopinath, N., S.L. Chadha, P. Jain, S. Shekhawat and R. Tandon. 1995. "An epidemiological study of coronary heart disease in different ethnic groups in Delhi urban population". *J Assoc Physicians India*, 43: 30–33.

Gupta, R., A. Misra, P. Pais, P. Rastogi and V.P. Gupta. 2005. "Correlation of regional cardiovascular disease mortality in India with lifestyle and nutritional factors". *Int J Cardiol*. June 21 (in press).

Goulding, A. et al. 1986. "Sodium and osteoporosis", in M.L. Wahlqvist and A.S. Truswell (eds.), *Recent Advances in Clinical Nutrition*. John Libby, London, pp. 99–108.

Harris, N. 2004. "Nutrition in Aging", in K. Mahan and S. Escott-Stump (eds.), *Krause's Food Nutrition and Diet Therapy*. 11th edition, W.B. Saunders Company, Philadelphia, pp. 318–337.

Heaney, R.P. 1987. "The role of nutrition in prevention and management of osteoporosis". *Clinical Obstetrics and Gynecology*, 50: 833–846.

Hennekens, C.H. et al. 1996. "Lack of effect of long-term supplementation with beta-carotene on the incidence of malignant neoplasms and cardiovascular disease". *New England Journal of Medicine*, 334: 1145–1149.

Institute of Medicine. 1998. "Dietary Reference Intakes for thiamin, riboflavin, niacin, vitamin B_6, folate, vitamin B_{12}, pantothenic acid, biotin and choline". National Academy Press, Washington.

National Nutrition Monitoring Bureau. 1999. "Report of Second Repeat Survey-Rural (1996–97)". National Institute of Nutrition, Hyderabad.

Omenn, G.S. et al. 1996. "Effects of a combination of beta-carotene and vitamin A on lung cancer and cardiovascular disease". *New Eng J of Med*, 334: 1150–1155.

Puri, S. 1999. "Dietary Antioxidants and Ageing: A Review", in Kalyan Bagchi and Seema Puri (eds.), *Diet and Ageing: Exploring Some Facets*. Society for Gerontological Research and HelpAge India.

—. 2001. "Nutritional Concerns of Older Persons", in Aabha Chaudhary (ed.), *Active Ageing in the New Millennium*. Anugraha, Delhi.

Sabate, J. 1999. "The contribution of vegetarian diets to health and disease: A paradigm shift?" *Am J Clin Nutr*, 78(3): 502S–507S.

Seddon, J.M. et al. 1994. "Dietary carotenoids, vitamins A, C, and E, and advanced age-related macular degeneration: Eye Disease Case-Control Study Group". *JAMA*, 272: 1413–1420.

Selhub, J. et al. 1993. "Vitamin status and intake as primary determinants of homocysteinemia in an elderly population". *JAMA*, 270: 2693–2698.

The Alpha-Tocopherol, Beta Carotene Cancer Prevention Study Group. 1994. "The effect of vitamin E and beta carotene on the incidence of lung cancer and other cancers in male smokers". *New England Journal of Medicine*, 330: 1029–1035.

World Health Organization. 2003. *World Health Report*.

World Health Organization. 1990. "Diet, nutrition and prevention of chronic diseases". *Tech Rep Ser*, 797: 1–204.

World Health Organization. 1999. *Development of food-based dietary guidelines for the Western Pacific*.

11 Nutrition and Health Policy

V.S. Natarajan

Ageing is a gradual process taking place over many decades. It has been repeatedly shown in studies involving animals that diet can have a significant influence on longevity and the ageing process. There are three types of ageing processes. "Normal ageing" includes inexorable and universal physiological changes that occur with ageing. "Usual ageing" includes age-related diseases, which result from the interaction between genetic, environmental and behavioral factors. "Successful ageing" includes modification of behavioral processes to achieve the best possible outcome to ageing.

Nutritional Requirements

As the ageing process progresses, a concomitant decline in organ function typically accompanies it. These changes in functionality might reasonably be expected to influence the nutrient needs of the individual.

Energy

There is no exact data about calorie requirement in the elderly in India. Calorie requirements decrease with age, due to low BMR and reduced physical activity, being about 25 per cent less than those of younger adults.

Protein

Total protein and lean body mass decline with age. A high protein diet may be less well digested and absorbed in the elderly as judged by a small increase in faecal nitrogen content in response to a protein load. RDA currently recommends 0.8–1 g protein.

Carbohydrate

Carbohydrate absorption may be slightly impaired with advanced age. Although there is no RDA for carbohydrates, 50 to 60 per cent of total calories should be from carbohydrates.

Fat

Fat digestion and absorption in the elderly is equivalent to that of young adults. Fat malabsorption in the elderly, when found, is often due to bacterial overgrowth of the small intestine. There is no RDA for total fat. However, it is widely accepted that 30 per cent of calories may be derived from fat.

Vitamins

Thiamin – there is no change in absorption; any deficiency is due to low intake. Riboflavin – there is no change in absorption or in tissue concentration. Ascorbic acid – it is adversely affected by smoking, medications, stress. Niacin – there is no change with age. Vitamin B_6 – decrease with age; RDA should be higher. Vitamin B_{12} – a low intake with impaired absorption is responsible for low levels of B_{12}; more vitamin B_{12} is needed.

Folic Acid

Marginal folate deficiency is associated with increased homocystine. Risk factor for IHD, stroke, PVD. Low folate is also linked to colon cancer and Alzheimer's disease.

Hyperhomocystinemia and Loss of Memory in the Elderly

An increased plasma homocysteine level has been reported to be a strong and independent risk factor for the development of dementia and Alzheimer's diseases. An open labelled study was conducted in elderly individuals having various grades of cognitive impairment. The homocysteine levels were estimated and the Gottfries Brane and Steen (GBS) Scale was administered on enrollment. The patients were then treated with a preparation called MCBM 69 containing three Homocysteine lowering vitamins viz. Methylcobalamin 500 mcg, Pyridoxine (Vit B_6) 3 mg and folic acid (Vit B_9) 1.5 mg. The tablets were administered twice daily for 6 months. The homocysteine levels were examined and the GBS scale readministered on completion of treatment at 6 months.

A total of 21 patients (13 males and 8 females) were enrolled in the study. The mean age was 75.86 + 1.91 years. The mean baseline GBS score was 15.05 + 1.53 and the mean baseline homocysteine level was 11.77 + 0198 micromols/L. 9 out of 21 patients had hyperhomocysteinemia. Following 6 months treatment with MCBM 69, an improvement in the GBS scale was noted in 71.43 per cent (15/21) of cases. Moreover, the mean GBS score reduced from 15.05 + 1.53 to 10.57 + 1.37 and the difference was statistically very highly significant (P 0.001). In 5 out of the 9 patients having hyperhomocysteinemia, the homocysteine levels normalized and in the others there was a significant fall. The mean homocysteine level on the completion of treatment reduced to 10.28 + 0.69 micromols/L.

In elderly patients with loss of memory, treatment with homocysteine lowering vitamins caused a reduction in the homocysteine levels and a definite improvement in the cognitive function. A trial in a larger sample of the population is warranted.

Vitamin D

Vitamin D is essential for the absorption of calcium and is more important for bone health. More vitamin D is needed. Older skin has reduced capacity to synthesis pre-vitamin D3. Declining kidney function result in impaired synthesis of active metabolities of vitamin D. Intake is frequently below the RDA.

Vitamin E

Vitamin E contains antioxidative properties which can help slow down the ageing process.

Vitamin D Deficiency Increase Risk of Prostate Cancer (Finland Study, 2004)

The etiology of cancer of the prostate remains unclear. The cause of prostate cancer is multifactorial, involving both genetic and environmental risk factors (age, race, geography, diet, hereditary factors). In Finland a study has been conducted to find out the association between vitamin D deficiency and prostate cancer and the following aspects were noted. Vitamin D deficiency may be an important cause in countries having seasonally low UV irradiation. A lack of vitamin D plays a role in the initiation, promotion, and progression of cancer. The action of vitamin D is due to its antiproliferative effect. High serum vitamin D levels delay the development of prostate cancer. Prevention: Vitamin D deficiency to be managed by dietary supplementation and by higher UV exposure.

Diet is a Nature's Poly Pill

A new poly pill was launched a few years back which can lower the risk of heart attack by 88 per cent and of stroke by 80 per cent in people over 55 years. The new poly pill is a combination of 6 drugs like statin, folic acid, aspirin and 3 other drugs. But this drug has its own side effects, ex: Aspirin induced gastritis. So this poly pill is not popular in Western countries. But one could get similar benefits if one included the following foods in their diet:

Table 11.1 ***Foods and Its Benefits***

What you should eat	*Benefits*
Soya (50 gm/day)	Heart and stroke risk cut by 45 per cent
Isabgol (15 gm/day)	Heart risk, blood sugar lowered.
Garlic (4 cloves/day)	Reduces plaque formation and heart risk
Fenugreek (25 gm/day)	Lowers cholesterol and blood sugar
Bengal gram (50 gm/day)	Lowers heart risk by 24 per cent.
Oat bran (25 gm/day)	Lowers heart risk by 27 per cent
Amla (2/day)	A powerful antioxidant

A Study on Nutritional Disorders and Nutrient Deficits in a Rural Community in Tamil Nadu Sponsored by Sandoz Foundation for Gerontological Research, Australia

In India 88 per cent of the elderly population live in rural area and 12 per cent live in urban areas. This study aims to identify common nutritional disorders and to look at the relationship between the social parameters and nutritional status in rural elderly people. This study will help to formulate a national plan to improve nutritional status of elderly people by enhancing the financial status, promoting health education and formulating good meal plans. The study was conducted in a rural elderly community consisting of ten villages surrounding Melmaruvathur, which is 91 km from Chennai. Eight hundred elderly people above 60 years were included.

A door to door survey was conducted by a social worker, who collected data on socio-economic and other related problems. All the elderly people were referred to Melmaruvathur for clinical, nutritional and biochemical examination. Anthropometry was used since it is an important method of assessing nutritional status in the elderly people. A thorough clinical examination was done by a research medical officer under the supervision of a geriatrician. The dietary patterns of all of the subjects were assessed with the help of a dietitian using questionnaire.

A three day recall data was collected from each individual. The raw equivalent of the cooked food consumed was computed and the nutritional value of raw foods consumed was calculated using the food composition table. The nutrient intake of the subjects was compared with the Recommended Daily Allowances (RDA) for Indians, given by the Indian Council of Medical Research (ICMR).

Results

The prevalence of underweight was high in this rural elderly community (55%), while obesity was uncommon (1.9%). It was found that 93.2 per cent of the elderly people studied had a low calorie intake. Ninety-eight per cent of the subjects had their protein intake less than ICMR recommended allowance. The average daily intake of protein was 24 G. The average intake of fat in the study was 18 G per day. Ninety-three per cent of the subjects had a low fat intake. There was a surplus of calcium intake in 33.5 per cent of the subjects. The reason may be due to moderate consumption of calcium rich cereal (ragi) and green leafy vegetables.

Table11.2 ***Mean Daily Nutrient Intake of the Elderly People***

Nutrients	*RDA of ICMR (1989)**		*Nutrient intake of elderly people studied*		
	Male	Female	Male (n=376) Mean	Female (n=424) Mean	Total(n=800) % of elderly people with low intake
Energy (kcal)	1760**	1350**	1019	850	93.2
Protein (g)	60	50	27	22	98.2
Calcium (mg)	400	400	394	337.6	66.5
Iron (mg)	28	30	14.5	12.8	93.5
Carotene (ug)	2400	2400	905.61	648.3	87.0
Thiamine (mg)	1.1	0.9	0.77	0.6	85.5
Riboflavin (mg)	1.4	1.1	0.50	0.4	98.2
Niacin (mg)	16	12.0	7.63	6.0	97.0
Vitamin C (mg)	40	40	41.71	28.9	79.0

Except calcium, the intake of all nutrients was low in this study. Socio-economic factors such as poverty, illiteracy, lack of nutritional knowledge and unfavourable domestic circumstances may have affected nutritional status.

Conclusion

Multiple nutrient deficiencies in the elderly are highly prevalent in the community, and even more so in rural areas. Extreme vitamin deficiency can cause irreversible organ damage. Given that it is difficult to make a diagnosis of sub-clinical nutrient deficiencies, supplementation should begin before signs appear.

Recommendations

- Imparting knowledge through media and multipurpose social workers.
- Nutrient supplementations should include more protein, B-complex, calcium and high fibre. Supply through public distribution service or domicilliary visit.

12 Elder Abuse and Adult Protection

Mala Kapur Shankardass

Elder abuse and neglect, despite denials from certain sources, are a not new phenomenon in India. As a subject worthy of serious academic inquiry and concerted action, it has begun to receive attention only at the turn of the 21st century, and with the rapidly growing numbers and proportions of older persons in the population gradually being acknowledged as a significant group having rights, requiring care, services and programmes to help them live a life of dignity and respect (Shankardass, 2003b). However, some significant commentaries and small scale studies on elder abuse and related issues conducted in the 1990s (Shah et al., 1995; Bambawale, 1996 and 1997; Kapoor, 1997; Shankardass, 1997; Prakash, 1998; Ushasree and Basha, 1999; Ramamurti and Jamuna, 1999; Jamuna and Padmasree, 2000) paved the way for greater academic and research interest.

In India, responsibility of taking care of older persons, supporting and protecting them traditionally has fallen on individuals in the family and the community. Yet, family and community are now also recognized as being responsible for elder abuse and neglect, though defining and identifying it is still controversial (Shankardass, 2004c). The predominant focus of limited public attention, available research, and academic interest has been on the abuse and neglect of older persons in the domestic and community settings, and there has been very little concern with abuse and neglect occurring within institutional settings (Shankardass, 2003b and 2004c). Perhaps because comparatively few older people are in institutions in India and those living there are to a large extent voiceless and powerless. The term 'institution' typically refers to a wide range of settings, such as hospitals, and long-term care facilities, which include nursing homes and homes for the aged.

Nonetheless, it is an emerging issue requiring due consideration and inquiry, especially as the need for institutional provisions for older people is growing. There is an increasing emphasis of the concept of social care (Puri, 2004a and b; Shankardass, 2004c).

The Issue of Elder Abuse and Neglect

The issue of abuse and neglect in India, as elsewhere in many other countries too, has been associated more with children and women. For older people, it is still underrecognized and insufficiently acknowledged. This is mainly due to an absence of valid statistics and systematic collection of facts related to the problem; limited studies; inadequate documentation (notwithstanding underreporting as well as the lack of conceptual and definitional clarity); a taboo on discussing the subject; and the consistent denial by family members that abuse takes place in their homes (Shankardass, 2003b). This is unlike the western countries where the issue has been recognized since the 1970s (Burston, 1975). For instance, in the USA, the problem has been identified from the mid-1970s, and since then it has been researched in an attempt to clarify the concept as well as to provide solutions to it. In Canada too, around this time it began to be recognized that while most Canadians live in comfort and with support provided by caring family members, there is a proportion of older adults who face exploitation and abuse (Novak, 1997). In fact, in 1990, a national survey conducted on the prevalence of elder abuse indicated that 1 in 25 people over the age of 65, living in the community suffered some form of abuse (Podnieks et al., 1990). In Britain and Europe recognition that older people may be subjected to abuse and neglect within their families as well as by outsiders and that socio-political and legislative action is required for combating it, dates from the mid-1980s with the seminal work of Mervyn Eastman (1984). In Australia, abuse and neglect of older people by family members began to be recognized by the late 1980s and soon there was a confirmation of it as a social, medical, and legal problem in both residential care and the community (Kurrle, 2003). In some of the developing countries of South and Latin America, since the 1990s, mistreatment of older persons has no longer been considered "a new issue" (Machado, 2001; Daichman et al., 2001; WHO/INPEA, 2002). In the developing countries of Asia, which are only recently recognized as ageing societies, concern with elder abuse and neglect has emerged only from the late 1990s or from the beginning of this century. Quite clearly, as demographic transitions are taking place in most countries and there are increases in the number of older people, greater emphasis is being brought to the concepts of successful ageing and this is prompting attention in the respective nations and in the world to the incidence, risk and vulnerabilities of older people for abuse and neglect.

In India, with the increase in the older population, defined as 60 years and above, currently almost 8 per cent of the total population, projected to be 142 million by 2020 from the 77 million as per the 2001 census, the issue of elder abuse and neglect can no longer be ignored. The National Policy on Older Persons has been in place since 1999, and the National Council for Older Persons has also been established. Elder abuse and neglect is a concern requiring action from the government and society. Further, India participated in the Second World Assembly on Ageing held in 2002 where the Madrid International Plan of Action on Ageing and the Political Declaration were adopted. the Plan of Action states that "Governments are also being encouraged to develop and fund a National comprehensive strategy and Agenda to prevent, detect and intervene in elder abuse" (Second World Assembly on Ageing, 2002). The concern for elder abuse and neglect requires immediate attention, policy response and societal interventions to reduce abusive environments and adopt combating strategies. It is important that there be more studies of elder abuse and neglect (though these are difficult to conduct) and attempts must be made to assess systematically the extent and nature of abuse in different parts of the country and also on a national level. It would be also meaningful for both government and society to recognize elder abuse not only as a social problem but also as a public health and legal issue (Shankardass, 2003a and b).

Prevalence and Incidence of Elder Abuse and Neglect in India

There are no reliable national level data in India on the prevalence and incidence of elder abuse and neglect. In fact to a large extent it is hidden by older people, their families and communities, as neither people nor government want to acknowledge, see, hear, or talk about this sort of behaviour, which is absolutely contradictory to the value system of compassion and support prevalent in Indian society. It is true that elder abuse and neglect are difficult to quantify as these occur in the privacy of the home, or in institutions, and reporting systems for elder abuse are almost absent in the country. There is no mandatory mechanism to report mistreatment, neglect, or abuse of older people in Indian society unlike in some western countries. Nonetheless, we may extrapolate that elder abuse in India, in all communities and across all sections of the society, is on the rise. Increasing media coverage, stories filed by journalists (Verma, 1996; Mitra, 1998; Paul, 1998), news reports in both print and electronic media (Menon, 1998; Martyris, 1999; Mehta, 2000), growing evidence from crime records, small scale, mainly qualitative, research studies, (Mahajan, 1992; Vaithi, 1996; Bambawale, 1996 and 1997; Prasad, 1997; Shankardass, 1997, 2002, 2004b; Jamuna, 1998; Ushasree and Basha, 1999; Prakash, 2004; Puri, 2004a and b) and NGO activities[1] directed towards addressing the multitude of issues related to the abuse make it clear that abuse and neglect of older people is emerging as a widespread serious problem. Testimony to its occurrence in some form or the other is also revealed in films made from time to time to reflect social reality, in literary stories and in some published biographical accounts (Shankardass, 2004b).

Evidence of growing incidence and prevalence is also being estimated by increases of old age homes and the demand for institutional care and care providers/givers from outside the family (Shankardass, 2003a and b). Elder abuse and neglect is seen to prevail among the different socio-economic groups, religious communities, and various regions, cutting across the rural-urban divide. It occurs at any educational level or at any development state. It seems to have a gender dimension with older women compared to older men seen to be vulnerable to it, but there have been increasing reports of abuse by older men.

Significantly a Report by United Nations Secretary-General Kofi Annan released at the Second World Assembly on Ageing, Madrid, Spain 8–12 April 2002 (United Nations, 2002) revealed that in India, in a sample of 1,000 older persons, 4 per cent claimed to be physically abused and in another smaller sample of 50 persons aged 70 years and over living in an urban area, 20 per cent said they had been neglected in their households. However, there are no systematic, methodologically sound studies to give a clear picture of the national level extent of the problem. As part of understanding the "Global Response to Elder Abuse" in 2001 a qualitative national study was commissioned by WHO-INPEA, which was conducted by HelpAge India. It was the first of its kind. It has certain limitations as it is based on focus groups of a sample population and it is exploratory.

It cannot be overstated that a database is necessary for policy, planning and practice to combat elder abuse. In India there is a need for statistics on the incidence and prevalence of elder abuse and neglect not only in private dwellings, but also in institutions and in society at large. There is a need to assess the nature and extent of abuse, and to identify who the perpetrators are. In conducting research to understand the magnitude of the problem it is essential to deal cautiously and methodologically with the underestimations of abuse, which arise due to a lack of reporting because victims and/or their families feel shame, guilt or fear. Incidence rates for elder abuse are difficult to assess. Even in countries where prevalence data on elder abuse exists there is no way of knowing whether the problem is getting better or worse. For intervention and educational strategies to be calibrated to meet current needs, it would be helpful to know the actual dimensions of the problem.

In order to understand the prevalence of elder abuse, the first step is towards clarification of definition and recognition of it in different settings and circumstances (Shankardass, 2004c). The need to develop parameters for identifying abuse requires concurrence. What kind of behaviour and action can be termed as abuse, given the variability of factors in providing care, such as poverty, lack of education and awareness of old age problems, economic and social constraints. Gender inequality and structural disadvantages add other aspects which require consideration. There is a need for dialogue, consciousness and societal response to tackle the issue (ibid.).

Understanding the prevalence of abuse may be linked to identifying the different systems in which this problem is addressed. For instance, if we define abuse within the parameters of social service system response, then the growth of agencies on ageing, such as not-for-profit community-based services to older adults and the increased provisions for adult protective service programmes mandated by the state can provide us with clues about its incidence and prevalence. Similarly if we regard abuse as a mental health issue, then growth and utilization of counselling centres, training programmes, stress relief interventions can provide indications about abuse and neglect. Similarly, if we view abuse as a legal issue, the response from the criminal justice system, the police, the courts, lawyers, judges, etc. become our guide to understanding the incidence and prevalence of abuse.

Identifying, Detecting and Defining Elder Abuse and Neglect

In public and academic discourses in India there is no consensus about the exact definition of 'elder abuse'. It is perceived in many different ways and it varies from the perspective of the families, care providers, legal functionaries, health providers, disciplinary specializations and that of older people themselves. However, academically, in gerontology it is a term which can be perceived under three broad areas, namely:

1. Neglect including isolation, abandonment and social exclusion.
2. Violation of human, legal and medical rights.
3. Deprivation of choices, decisions, status, finances and respect.

In Indian society elder abuse is often camouflaged by people, using other terms considered to be less severe, for instance, neglect, abandonment, disrespect, maltreatment, threats, emotional blackmail, loss of dignity, or exploitation. The public and academics often assert that abuse is a very strong word, one generally equated with very violent physical behaviour, which does not happen in our families or communities (Shah et al., 1995; WHO/INPEA, 2002; Shankardass, 2003a and b). Yet, there are increasing reports of physical assault, excessive restraint, murders, and culpable homicide not amounting to murder, crime and violence against older persons in police records, media coverage and public narratives. However, detection of elder abuse and neglect is notoriously difficult, often complicated by denial by the concerned individual and the caretaker. As my research with older people indicates problems arise in obtaining an accurate and objective history of abuse and neglect. Often symptoms of abuse are similar to physiological ageing of individuals and detection and identification of abuse is further made difficult by victims being reluctant to admit and report abuse. Fear of abandonment by the carer, reprisal, institutionalization, shame and avoidance of embarrassment contribute significantly to the underdiagnosis and the underreporting of elder abuse and neglect by the victims. Non-confessions by the perpetrators, unwillingness of witnesses to testify and unclear evidence adds to the difficulties in identifying and detecting the occurrence of elder abuse and neglect.

Based on research conducted by individuals and organizations, complaints lodged with NGOs, police records, and media reports, my analysis as a researcher and activist in this field indicates that some of the common forms of elder abuse experienced with the action of family members (spouse, children and other relatives) acquaintances (friends, neighbours, servants, service providers) and unknown people (robbers, murderers) in the country are:

- Material exploitation – using money, assets, property without allowing control and giving benefits of that to the ageing owner.
- Financial deprivation – not letting the older person have enough resources to meet daily needs and maintain adequate quality of life.

- 'Property grabbing' – making the older person homeless, asset less.
- Isolation – cutting off the older person from family, social, and community activities.
- Abandonment – compelling or leaving the older person to live in an institution, referred to as 'ashram' or old age home.
- Verbal humiliation – being insulting, rude, insensitive, disrespectful and adopting ageist attitudes toward the older person.
- Emotional and psychological torment – giving threats, generating fear in the mind, increasing insecurity, inducing stress and strain, exposing to humiliating behaviour and breaking the confidence of the older person.
- Placing older persons' health at risk with poor or lack of care – not taking into account older persons disabilities and frailty, giving insufficient and non-nutritional food, not being responsive to diseases and illnesses of the older person, not assisting in seeking adequate and timely medical care and not providing sufficient care.

In Indian society, there is a tendency of dismissing the elder abuse cases that do come to light as a domestic issue, an internal matter of concerned individuals not to be addressed publicly with a multidimensional approach and an understanding of the underlying causes. Further to that is the belief, that many situations of neglect, deprivation, and marginalization are the normal consequence of ageing. In addition structural inequalities prevailing in society, such as low wages, high unemployment, poor health services, gender discrimination, lack of educational opportunities and limited awareness of ageing issues contribute to the vulnerability of older people, and constitute abuse and neglect by families, their communities, and society. Significantly, individual and family predictors based on health, personality, availability of resources, etc. along with societal and cultural factors, such as land rights, property and inheritance systems, social construction of gender and age, that place older women and the disabled at risk, as well as issues arising from social change because of migration, urbanization, modernization, technological development and environmental pressures of space are all seen to impact elder abuse and neglect.

Old and New Dimensions

The incidence of elder abuse in the country is not new. Generational conflicts resulting in interpersonal violence manifested in films, plays and creative literature are timeless. Some narratives of older people indicate the different forms of abuse (Shankardass, 2004b). Use of old age homes by the 'needy' elderly to pass their last days either as a last resort when for various reasons the family support system has broken down, or for seeking solace while disengaging from family and social concerns has a long history (Shankardass, 2000). The first old age home documented in literature was set up as far back as the early 18th century. Since then many more have been added. There is no current exact data on the number of old age homes as many are not registered. But a directory of registered old age homes in the first edition, published in 1995, listed 500 homes. The second edition which came out in 1998 had a list of about 700 homes. The revised edition brought out in 2002 lists 995 homes in 25 states and union territories of India (Shankardass, 2000).

However, the types or categories of abuse visible today in society are many more than have been observed in the past given the growing understanding of human rights, gender equality and ageism. For instance, the treatment being meted out to ageing women, particularly widows, is beginning to be critically considered in terms of property rights, their role in family and society, their disengagement, the lack of suitable provisions for leisure, recreation and their participation in household and work activities (Shankardass, 1999). Also the requirement for specialized care of older people by care givers is being viewed in terms of the burden and stress placed on the care-giver, and the suppression, accessibility to services, need for long term care, and the fulfilment of social and medical needs of the older person (Shankardass, 2003a, b and c). There is an increasing emphasis on addressing the issue by going beyond the earlier concerns of neglect and deprivation in domestic settings and placing the concerns of the elderly population in international discourses on rights, duties, and responsibilities.

Caring Services

Increasingly caring is being put into a service context, as concern with age-related diseases, for instance Alzheimer's and other forms of dementia, locomotive and chronic disabilities, grows. The need for training of care givers and bringing under scrutiny the care they provide are challenges beginning to be faced (Puri, 2004a and b; Shankardass, 2003b). Increasing number of studies are identifying care giver stress as a risk factor for elder abuse and neglect (Padamsree, 1991; Jamuna, 1997 and 1999, Puri, 2004b) and there is growing awareness of the need for training programmes for care givers, as they play a vital role in the prevention of abuse and neglect. Gendered aspects of abuse in terms of risks and vulnerabilities are also being recognized, as are the differences between receiving and giving care and control and ownership of property. Difficulties in accessing and utilizing services are also considered as vulnerabilities to elder abuse and neglect. While varied experiences of ageing are acknowledged, the need for the establishment of new services, for instance, day care centres, counselling units, rehabilitation services and respite care can not be understated in order to reduce the risk of elder abuse and neglect. The significance of religious organizations in playing a critical role in the prevention of elder abuse through fostering public awareness and providing services for families at risk of abusing also needs due consideration. How effective they can be in treatment intervention needs to be explored as they do occupy an important place in the lives of people in India.

For a long time abuse of older people was seen to be linked with negative stereotypes and attitudes (Bambawale, 1996 and 1997). These result in prejudices against older people and increase their risk of abuse and neglect. A social response is necessary to change negative attitudes about ageing and thereby to decrease the incidents of elder abuse and neglect. Media role and NGO participation in this direction becomes crucial. They can facilitate partnerships between young and old generations. An innovative action has been undertaken by HelpAge India through their initiative of 'Adopt a Granny' programme which fosters ties between school children and old, isolated, lonely people in the family, community, day care centres and old age homes and involves education initiatives centred around reducing abuse and neglect of older people in society. Another illustration of innovative initiatives taken by the NGO sector is that in some cities there are "friendly visitor" programmes where young adults or older able adults visit older people once or a few times per week and assist them in mundane household activities. These are becoming popular not only in big cities such as Delhi and Bangalore, but also in small towns.

The emerging emphasis on elder abuse in the country is thus focused on individual, familial and societal factors linked as they are to increasing longevity, feminization of ageing, old age-related diseases, processes of social change and wider problems of persistent poverty, unemployment, migration, urbanization, limited and inadequate social security provisions, unawareness of legal entitlements, limited protective legislations, lack of response from the medical community and families (Shankardass, 2003b). There is a recognition of these and many other factors, such as widowhood, financial dependence, assistance and support in daily activities, being a stressed out care giver, a demanding care-receiver, too little or too much of joint living, lonely living, etc., which put the older persons in vulnerable and disadvantaged positions in society due to age-discriminatory attitudes, systems and environments. Thus, many hypotheses can be offered as explanations for elder abuse and neglect but it would be best to have an integrated perspective which includes aspects of the care givers burden, stress, pathology and learned violence along with aspects of the victim, such as excessive dependency or certain personality traits and ongoing environmental stressors, such as limited space, economic resources, health, etc.

Impact on Older People

It is also important and useful to pay attention to another significant aspect that has generally been overlooked, which is the impact of elder abuse on older people. As my preliminary research indicates, mistreatment of older victims is seen to cause a range of long-term physical and psychological health problems, including permanent physical damage; medication and alcohol dependency; lowered immune system response; chronic eating disorders and malnutrition; self-harm or self-neglect; depression; fearfulness and chronic anxiety; suicidal tendencies; and death. These observations reflect another dimension of elder abuse and neglect, that is, older people themselves can be abusive. They may abuse themselves through self-neglect, or they may abuse members of their families or communities. My research with families caring for older people indicates that such incidences are not uncommon, but they have not been given adequate attention, or a theoretical or interventional focus. It is thus imperative that older people be seen in the context of their family, community and political environment and both the causes of abuse as well as its effects are recognized and dealt with.

While the symptoms of being a victim can be helpful in detecting abuse and neglect, interventions are also required to improve the quality of life of older people. Reaching out to affected older people, the victims of abuse and neglect, becomes extremely difficult given their situation. Also, detecting abuse and neglect at this advanced stage creates its own limitations by confusing the cause with the effect and vice versa. The remedies become extremely problematic and it presents challenges to developing and implementing a strategy for taking a comprehensive approach to elder abuse and neglect.

Institutional Abuse and Legal Aspects

The increasing number of long-term care institutions and residential complexes being established in all parts of the country makes the incidence of elder abuse in domestic settings more visible and increases the risk of older people to institutional abuse, though no systematic assessments have been made of the prevalence and incidence of such abuse. In fact institutional abuse is seldom considered a concern, although it merits attention especially in terms of the liability of those who organize and run institutions/old age homes with an obligation to care for the residents. The negligence in caring, dissatisfaction with care giving and ill treatment experienced by older persons in institutions has no doubt so far been sparingly documented (Rao and Devi Prasad, 1996; Rathod, 2000; Shankardass, 2003b) but the fact that it occurs should be enough to initiate action to prevent and combat abuse in these circumstances. Detecting and reporting elder abuse in institutions is made difficult by the fact that those using these provisions are generally most frail and vulnerable. However incidences of abuse can be reported by families especially when occurring in hospital settings but due to an absence of a mandatory reporting system, it does not happen in practice due to fear of non-cooperation from the staff involved. Besides, there is no clear definition of institutional abuse which can delineate what elder abuse is and how it is to be measured, thus limiting the input towards preventive measures.

My preliminary research on some of the senior citizen residential complexes indicates that while various safety and security steps are being taken to make older people comfortable in these dwellings, certain harm, inflicted due to clashes of personality and other differences, cannot be ruled out as instigating crime and violent behaviour towards older people. Moreover, there is very little awareness about older peoples' rights and responsibilities and there is an almost negligible awareness about the fact that institutions involved in caring for older persons do have legal liability and obligations to perform their task through the Indian Contract Act 1872 and the Law of "Torts" whereby for any mistreatment and failure in caring, a civil suit can be filed against the management of the institution for the breach in contract to care, even though there might not be a written contract and damages can be claimed for the wrong done (Shankardass, 2003b). Institutions, which are in the business of caring for older persons, have not so far been brought under legal purview, but there is a need to take seriously the provision in the Indian Penal Code under which, breach of contract may amount to criminal liability (Bakshi, 2000). However problems in implementing these measures arise from the fact that it is difficult to conduct proper investigations and to prove the intent of abuse and maltreatment, and this may stop the older person from taking a decision to report the abuse.

Government Response to Elder Abuse

The National Policy on Older Persons formulated in January 1999 by the Ministry of Social Justice and Empowerment does not refer specifically to the incidence and prevalence of elder abuse, but does acknowledge, as a concern, emerging "pressures and fissures in living arrangements of older persons" as a consequence of the demographic (ageing of the population) in the country. The policy under the section on implications of demographic trends, which are seen at the macro and the household level, stresses that the family ties in India are strong with an overwhelming majority of older persons living with their sons, or supported by them, and also that working couples find the presence of old parents emotionally bonding and of great help in managing the household and caring for children. It nonetheless acknowledges that due to the operation of several forces, the position of a large number of older persons has become vulnerable. They cannot take for granted that their children will be able to look after them when they need care in old age, especially in view of the longer life span, implying an extended period of dependency and higher costs to meet health and other needs (Para 10).

Further, the policy document outlines: "Much higher costs of bringing up and educating children and pressures for gratification of their desires affects transfer of share of income for the care of parents." In understanding the changes in values and life styles which impact the lives of older persons negatively, the Policy refers to shortage of space in dwellings in urban areas and high rents whereby migrants prefer to leave their parents in their native place. It further elaborates, "Changing roles and expectations of women, their concept of privacy and space, desire not to be encumbered by caring responsibilities of old people for long periods, career ambitions, and employment outside the home implies considerably reduced time for care giving. Also, adoption of small family norm by a growing number of people implies availability of fewer care givers especially since in an increasing number of families, daughters, too, are fully occupied, pursuing their educational or work career". The concern in the policy is more visible with regard to the older women as attention is brought to their greater vulnerability as single persons since few persons are willing to take care of non-lineal relatives and particularly in case of widows who have no independent source of income, do not own assets and are totally dependent (Para 11).

Adult Protective Legislations

The government maintenance of old parents by children is a crucial issue and the Hindu Adoption and Maintenance Act, 1956 secures the rights of maintenance to the parents by the children, being applicable to both, sons and daughters, married or unmarried. The law relating to Muslims and other religious groups is not codified in India but the position regarding them is substantially the same. It is contained in the Code of Criminal Procedure, 1973, (even though the provision is really of a civil nature) in Section 125 (1) (2) which recognizes the right of parents without any means to be supported by their children having sufficient means. Thus there is a comprehensive statutory provision as to maintenance which is not confined to persons of any particular community (Shankardass, 2003b).

However, "maintenance" under Section 125 of the Code of Criminal Procedure, 1973 has not been defined, which gives leeway to the 'fair' completion of the case and suitable grant of maintenance for maintaining an adequate and appropriate standard of living as per the status of the old parent. While in settlement of some disputes liberal interpretation of maintenance has been adopted in the courts (Bakshi, 2000) with not being confined to food, clothing and shelter only, but including expenses of medical attendance also, the questions of justice and equity remain disputed even though the provision is intended to exclude destitution and vagrancy. In addition are the issues of complex, delayed and lengthy procedures which come in the way of giving relief and combating abuse. In developing preventive strategies, mechanisms to regulate care and monitor it in the family, community, and institutional settings, is necessary. Which programmes and initiatives can be undertaken requires an understanding within which they can operate. What measures need to be adopted from the social service, health, and criminal justice perspectives, require definition and debate.

Attempts to address these problems are made in the National Policy on Older Persons whereby it is stated that to simplify the procedure, provide speedy relief, lay down the machinery for processing cases and define the rights and circumstances in a comprehensive manner the states will be encouraged to pass legislations for securing the right to maintenance for parents so that they do not face abandonment and acute neglect (Para 32). Two states of India have already taken the initiative in this direction and a few others are in the process of framing their legislation. The policy statement recommends other states to follow suit.

The Himachal Pradesh Legislative Assembly passed the Himachal Pradesh Maintenance of Parents and Dependents Bill, 1996 which introduces a simple procedure for parents being ignored by their children to be given maintenance. It allows for the cases to be disposed of promptly, bringing justice and relief to older persons without loss of time, making it obligatory for errant wards to take care of their aged parents. The Government of Maharashtra also prepared a Bill along similar lines and the Government of Goa has a proposal for initiating action in this regard. Recently, the central government and the Delhi Government have taken up the exercise of reviewing appropriate legislations to protect and safeguard older people's rights and interests. Unfortunately most other state governments have not given serious thought to legal interventions for safeguarding the interests of older persons, but then the implementation of the National Policy has been slow since its formulation. Nonetheless some states do have other general statutory provisions which can be used by older persons under certain conditions. For instance, the Madhya Pradesh Government initiated the Madhya Pradesh Act No. 26 of 1976[2] which provides legal aid and legal advise to weaker sections including older people subject to fulfilling other eligibility criteria. This Act seeks to bring the system of justice within the reach of weaker sections of the population.

Role of Legal Interventions

While legal interventions are a powerful tool in addressing elder abuse issues, it does raise other pertinent questions about the rights of older persons with regard to those involved with care. These questions are critical and arouse doubt whether new legislations will be more effective since legal interventions are not often sought by the concerned party. A more fundamental concern relates to understanding what prevents people from using available legislations. Are criminal prosecutions appropriate when the perpetrators of abuse could be victims of their circumstances, for instance, maybe facing poverty, or experiencing excessive stress in caring for the old parents? Should criminalization of abuse and neglect as a combating strategy be encouraged or avoided? It also relates to another dimension that often notion of abuse is not conceptualized in legal terms by those involved, a phenomenon common to many countries (Phillipson and Biggs, 1995). Experiences from the West, where review of measures adopted has been taking place, suggest that it is much more productive and fruitful to treat elder abuse as a social service concern than to deal with it as a new area of criminal behaviour (Formby, 1992). For instance in the US it is seen that while adult protective legislation has given support to vulnerable older persons, in the absence of supportive services, legislation can do more harm than good (Phillipson and Biggs, 1995).

In the case of India, where we still believe that the sanctity of family ties and bonding prevails, and instances of abusive behaviour by the caregiver is seen more in the context of structural and societal factors, that is, for instance, in terms of poverty, financial and spatial constraints, or being unable to care due to ignorance and stress reaction, the fear of apprehension and punishment will not have much meaning, nullifying the impact of legislations. However, as some recent reports, especially those pertaining to inheritance and property disputes, or due to acute financial and physical dependence indicate that abuse may be deliberate with the intent to harm the victim physically, emotionally, materially or even sexually, then it would be advisable to initiate criminal investigation. The case should be dealt with criminal proceedings within the channels of the criminal justice system.

The policy statement under the 'Principal areas of intervention and action strategies' notes that "old persons have become soft targets for criminal elements." It gives a hope of combating the problem by providing under the section on 'Protection of Life and Property' a promise for the introduction of a clause in the Indian Penal Code which shall protect older persons from domestic violence, specifically in the context of deprivation of their rights of inheritance, occupancy, etc. The policy statement also refers to assisting voluntary organizations and associations of older persons in providing protective services and help to older persons through helpline services, legal aid and other measures. Further it directs the police to keep a vigil on older couples and more specifically on old single persons especially those living alone, and to strengthen the neighbourhood watch system.

However, the criminal justice and legal system in the country does not have a definite response to elder abuse as it has not clearly defined elder abuse and neglect nor does it see it as an issue of concern to law enforcement. However, in recent years increases in crime, generally finance and property related crimes against older persons is putting pressure on the criminal justice and legal system to respond and protect older people. There is public consensus that law enforcement agencies must play an active role in identifying and prosecuting those who prey on older people. As a response to public demand and as a part of the preventive criminal justice programme in many major cities and metropolitan towns the law enforcement organizations have issued handouts that include information on how to safeguard against elder abuse and crime. In some cities police are disseminating crime prevention tips for older adults on a regular basis. Also community policing initiatives are being developed that target prevention of elder abuse especially those that rise to the level of a crime. Police patrol residential colonies with a higher percentage of older people regularly, and visit senior citizens living alone to deter servants or other service providers from indulging in any criminal activity against older people. In some cities 'Helpline' services senior citizens or their well-wishers can access quick help in times of need. In Chennai such service has been launched in conjunction with the Tamil Nadu Police force. The helpline operates from the office of the Commissioner of Police. A social worker and a psychologist are available at the other end of the line. Just by dialing 1253, a toll-free number, people can get advice on care and other aspects. The helpline staff also acts on cases referred by other people, making referrals to hospitals for healthcare and counselling for elders having family problems. Financial counselling and legal assistance are also a part of their work.

These programmes are developing primarily in urban areas where the risk of crime is seen to be greater for older people. There is yet, no national elder abuse public awareness campaigns although increasing numbers of older people are being manipulated into handing over their assets. Few NGOs and voluntary organizations have taken up the task of educating older people on financial and other forms of abuse and have developed partnerships with legal functionaries and chartered accountants to issue guidelines for being proactive in the prevention of financial abuse of older people. A few noteworthy illustrations of such practices are Development, Welfare and Research Foundation, a voluntary organization operating from Delhi, which conducts frequent awareness programmes for improving quality of life of older people; HelpAge India public lecture programmes; and in Mumbai programmes of Dignity, Dialogue and Harmony also contribute in this direction.

These organizations are working towards building directories of helpful resources and websites. They are establishing telephone helplines to educate callers about the abuse of older persons and about the resources available to them, and to refer them to help agencies. They are offering awareness and education programmes in a number of settings. Community development programmes that address needs and concerns of older persons help to raise awareness and educate about abuse. In many other cities my research indicates that seminars are given to older adults in senior centres, retirement association offices, community and religious centres where older people may congregate. Interviews with older people reveal the benefits of such discussions which empower them to recognize and avoid financial exploitation and other forms of abuse.

Health Sector Response

Response from the health community to elder abuse is of very recent origin since Geriatrics as a specialization is gradually making inroads in primary health care and community health programmes. The past initiatives have been limited, fragmented and lacking in direction. A majority of the problems older persons experience occur in the community and, while a primary care approach may be one of the possible approaches pursued to improve the quality of life, little attention has been paid to strengthening the role of the health provider in detection and management of elder abuse. No doubt, detection of elder abuse is very difficult, being a sensitive issue, and it requires not only tact and discretion in dealing and managing it, but also involvement of several professionals from the medical, nursing, social work, rehabilitation fields, etc. But health care professionals can be important contributors of care for older people who have been abused. For one, the involvement of these formal care givers helps in preventing further abuse and neglect. However, health professionals require education and training to deal with the issue and an important step lies in changing their attitudes and beliefs about ageing and violence in general. Thus education of medical and health professionals is a critical component of knowledge and skill development. It provides the necessary foundation upon which to offer services. It is encouraging that certain national level initiatives in preparing training modules for health professionals have been undertaken with the support of the World Health Organization (WHO). Also those involved with promoting geriatric medicine in the country, through educational materials, seminars and workshops, are encouraging health professionals to undertake a thorough and compassionate assessment of older patients and to make it the foundation for planning the care of older people. Some of the parameters being recommended in the clinical assessment of older patients are, namely, medical and social concerns, living situation, family composition, social supports, sensory losses, financial resources, vulnerability, activity level, mental health, participation in activities of daily living and instrumental activities of daily living, etc. (Rosenblatt and Natarajan, 2002).

The contribution of the physician or the primary health care provider in preventing elder abuse can be effective in several ways beginning with an assessment of the older person's physical and mental capacity, an assessment of the general quality of care, an assessment of the relationship of the older person with the care provider, an assessment of the abusers' problems and moving on to becoming a counsellor and enabler for liaison with the police or social worker when the older person is incapable of or does not want to accept help. The role of the physician may also involve interaction with other family members and relatives. The physician can advise institutionalization if abuse cannot be prevented at home. For the health professionals to be effective it would be essential to develop resource materials which would assist them in detecting and preventing the abuse of older persons. This could include screening tools to identify abusive and potentially abusive situations, protocols for referral and intervention, and a training resource kit for service providers.

Recognize 'The Hidden Patient'

It is also important to recognize the 'care-giver burden' which leads to a variety of physical, emotional, social and financial stresses for the care giver. As a preventive strategy for elder abuse it is important to recognize the 'hidden patient', the care-giver, to whose needs attention of the health care worker must also go. Prolonged stress of caring ultimately affects the well-being and living conditions of the older person often resulting in neglect and abuse by the care giver. Quite clearly, care giver stress is a risk factor for elder abuse and neglect and education and training programmes for formal and informal care givers play a vital role in prevention. It would be useful to build care giver support groups which could be a resource, assisting in the care of the older adult. Such programmes have already started in some of the urban areas of the country, particularly as a response to deal with the care of Alzheimer's and dementia patients, and also with terminal illnesses.

These care giver support groups typically offer mutual support, stress reduction and work towards problem solving strategies.

Conclusion

Quite clearly, understanding and dealing with elder abuse and neglect requires an urgent societal response from social, legal and public health perspectives. There is a pressing need for consolidated progressive action by social scientists, policy makers, administrators, social workers, legal and public health specialists, and older persons themselves in tackling the existing problems of defining on a theoretical and empirical front is important, as not all of the situations characterized internationally as abuse fit neatly into legal categories or into the socio-cultural context of Indian society. Many a time acts of abuse are regarded as normal behaviour given the variations in perceptions of roles, literacy levels, and social economic status. Consequently, more effort has to go into understanding the underlying causes of abuse, identifying risk factors and developing appropriate public health interventions.

A commitment at the national level towards research, education, and action, on behalf of India's abused and neglected older adults which is showing signs of increasing, has to be nurtured. Public awareness of the abuse of older people has to be raised constantly and people sensitized to the problem whereby they not only work towards reducing abusive situations and environments but also offer support to victims and also encourage them to seek help. Public education programmes and campaigns against abuse and neglect have to be geared towards those who are in a position to recognize abuse when it occurs. Many more national, regional, and local conferences, as well as meetings directed toward professionals, the public, and seniors themselves should be organized to address the multitude of issues related to the abuse and neglect of older adults. A wealth of educational materials is being produced and strategies for prevention of elder abuse are being advocated from the local to the national levels. These need larger resources for dissemination and continuous government support to fund innovative responses to the problem.

There is a need for more attention to adult protection legislation, along with advances in the creation of protocols for detection, intervention, and programming. On the one hand increased awareness about legislation already in place to protect the interests of older persons has to be promoted. On the other hand, difficulties being experienced in using legal measures for relief from abuse have to be addressed. There is hesitation on the part of older persons to sue their family members and institutional managers for breach of contract. Empowering the older persons to demand and have their needs fulfilled within the human rights framework is a challenge for societies to take up. The elderly of today and those of the future deserve a life of dignity and well-being. Ageing is to be celebrated.

Notes

1. Many non-government regional and local levels, for instance, HelpAge India; Age Care India; Development, Welfare and Research Foundation; Centre for the Welfare of the Aged; Society for Gerontological Research; OutrEach; Dignity Dialogue; Heritage Trust; etc. have been working for the cause of older persons and promoting awareness of abuse.
2. The MP Act No. 26 of 1976 has a Hindi title which is *The Madhya Pradesh Samaj ke Kamjor Vargon ke Liye Vidhik Sahayata*, voluntary and charitable organizations working at national, *Tatha Vidhik Salah Adhiniyam*. When translated into English it means that it supports the Madhya Pradesh weaker sections legal aid and legal advice provisions.

References

Bakshi, P.M. 2000. "Senior citizens and the law", in P.C. Bhatla (ed.), *Lecture Series in Geriatrics*. Health Care Promotion Trust, New Delhi: National Institute of Primary Health Care, p. 415.

——. 2000. "Homes for the aged-legal aspects", in P.C. Bhatla (ed.), *Lecture Series in Geriatrics*. Health Care Promotion Trust, New Delhi: National Institute of Primary Health Care, pp. 416–417.

Burston, G.R. 1975. "Granny battering". *British Medical Journal*, 3(6), p. 592.

Bambawale, Usha. 1996. "Abuse of the Aged", in V. Kumar (ed.), *Ageing: Indian Perspectives and Global Scenario*. New Delhi: All India Institute of Medical Sciences, pp. 298–302.

——. 1997. "The abused elderly". *Indian Journal of Medical Research*, 106, October, pp. 389–395.

Daichman, L., O. Guido, S. Aguas and M. Bertone. 2001. "Report on Elder Abuse in Argentina". WHO/INPEA.

Eastman, Mervyn. 1984. "Old Age Abuse". London: Age Concern England.

Formby, W.A. 1992. "Should elder abuse be decriminalized? A justice system perspective". *Journal of Elder Abuse and Neglect*, 4(4), pp. 121–30.

Jamuna, D. 1997. "Stress dimensions among caregivers of the elderly". *The Indian Journal of Medical Research*, Special Issue: *Aging in India*, 106, pp. 381–387.

——. 1999. "Stress among caregivers: Do interventions help?" *Indian Journal of Gerontology*.

Jamuna, D. and V. Padmasree. 2000. "Psycho-social profiles of abused elderly". *Indian Journal of Gerontology*.

Kapoor, P. 1997. "Elderly Abuse: Some Counseling Tips". *Research and Development Journal*, 3(3), pp. 13–23.

Kurrle, Susan. 2003. 'The Systems of Prevention and Detection of Abuse in Australia', Symposists' Papers, Invited Symposia on Elder Abuse, Executive Editor, Toshio Tatara, Tokyo International Forum, Japan.

Machado, Laura. 2001. "National Report on Elder Abuse in Brazil". WHO/INPEA.

Mahajan, A. 1992. "Social dependency and abuse of the elderly", in P. Krishnan and K. Mahadevan (eds.), *The Elderly Population in Developed and Developing World*. New Delhi: B.R. Publishing Corporation, pp. 414–423.

Martyris, Nina. 1999. "Help is just a phone-call away". *The Times of India*, February 28.

Mehta, Rajul. 2000. "Exploitation and neglect are indicators of abuse". *The Times of India*, January 15.

Menon, Leela. 1998. "In forward-looking Kerala, there is no future for the aged". *Indian Express*, Special Report.

Mitra, Sumit. 1998. "Old parents unlovingly yours". *India Today*, July 13.

Novak, M. 1997. *Aging and Society: A Canadian Perspective*. Third Edition, Toronto: ITP Nelson.

Paul, Sumita. 1998. "With a little help from friends". *The Sunday Times of India*, April 5.

Padmasree, V. 1991. "A Study of Incidence of Elder Abuse and Some Factors Related to Abuse". Unpublished Master Thesis, S.V. University, Tirupati.

Phillipson, Chris and Simon Biggs. 1995. "Elder abuse: A critical overview", in Paul Kingston and Bridget Penhale (eds.), *Family Violence and the Caring Professions*. London: Macmillan Press, p. 199.

Podnieks, E., K. Pillemer, J. Nicholson, T. Shillington and A. Frizzel. 1990. "National Survey on Abuse of the Elderly in Canada. Toronto", Ontario: Ryerson Polytechnic Institute.

Prakash, I.J. 1998. "Issues in mental health and psychological well being of older persons", in M. Desai and S. Raju (eds.), *Gerontological Social Work in India*. Delhi: B.R. Publishing Corp., pp. 185–203.

Prasad, B. Devi. 1997. "Elder abuse and neglect: A review of research and programmes", paper presented at the National Seminar on Globalization and the Ageing: Implications for Gerontological Social Work, organized by Tata Institute of Social Sciences and Family Welfare Agency, Mumbai, December 22–24.

Puri, Kiran. 2004a. "Preventing and Managing Neglect of Older People: The Importance of Reducing Burden of Care in Metropolitan Cities", paper presented at the National Seminar on Abuse of the Elderly, Thiruvananthapuram, November 29–30.

——. 2004b. "Reducing Burden of Care of the Elderly", paper presented at the XXXth All India Sociological Conference, Gorakhpur, December 28–30.

Ramamurti, P.V. and D. Jamuna. 1999. "Elder Abuse in the Indian Context". *Indian Journal of Gerontology.*

Rao, K. Visweswara and B. Devi Prasad. 1996. 'Attitudes of the youth and the middle aged people towards the elderly: A comparative study', paper presented at the National Workshop on Elder Abuse, organized by the Centre for the Welfare of the Aged (CEWA), Madras, March 16–17.

Rathod, Kishore. 2000. "Home alone and in pain". *Mid-Day*, March 2, pp. 1–2.

Rosenblatt, D.E. and V.S. Natarajan (eds.), 2002. *Primer on Geriatric Care: A Clinical Approach to the Older Patient*. Cochin: Printer's Castle.

Second World Assembly on Ageing, Plan of Action and Political Declaration, Madrid, Spain, 2002.

Shah, Gita, Rosamma Veedon and Sabiha Vasi. 1995. "Elder abuse in India". *Journal of Elder Abuse and Neglect* 6(3 and 4), pp. 101–108.

Shankardass, Mala Kapur. 1997. "The plight of older women: Victims of domestic violence", in K. Bagchi (ed.), *Elderly Females in India, their Status and Suffering.* New Delhi: Society for Gerontological Research and HelpAge India, pp. 79–88.

——. 1998. Key Note Address 'Challenges of the Changing Socio–Economic and Psychological Status of the Aged', delivered at the Regional Conference organized by HelpAge India, Chandigarh, January 21.

——. 1999. 'The Changing Social Role of Older Women', paper presented at the Symposium Challenges for the Family, Society and the Individual at International Conference on Women's Health–Nations Gain, TSAO Foundation, Singapore, July.

——. 2000a. "Societal Responses". *Seminar* 488, April.

——. 2000b. "Women and Ageing in South East Asia". WHO/SEARO.

——. 2002. "Situation and Voices: The Older Poor and Excluded in South Africa and India". *Population and Development Strategies Series* 2, UNFPA, New York.

——. 2003a. "Ageing Women and Abuse: Concerns and Need for Action". DWARF Research Brief, New Delhi: Development, Welfare and Research Foundation, Monograph, April.

——. 2003b. "Combating Elder Abuse in India: An Emerging Social, Legal and Public Health Concern", in *Understanding the Early Detection and Early Intervention in Elder Abuse in Developed and Developing Countries and Efforts to Develop Measures for Combating Elder Abuse in Asian Countries: A Status Report.* Symposists' Papers, Executive Editor, Toshio Tatara Tokyo International Forum, Japan.

——. 2003c. "Concerns for Ageing Women in India", in *BOLD, Quarterly Journal of the International Institute on Ageing* (United Nations - Malta), May, 13[3].

——. 2004a. "The Study of Ageing", in Ashish Bose and Mala Kapur Shankardass (eds.), *Growing Old in India: Voices Reveal and Statistics Speak*. B.R. Publishing House, New Delhi.

——. 2004b. "Voices Reveal", in Ashish Bose and Mala Kapur Shankardass (eds.), *Growing Old in India: Voices Reveal and Statistics Speak*. B.R. Publishing House, New Delhi.

——. 2004c. "Understanding Prevalence of Elder Abuse and Models to Prevent it", paper presented at the National Seminar on Abuse of the Elderly, Thiruvananthapuram, November 29–30.

The National Policy on Older Persons. Government of India, Ministry of Social Justice and Empowerment, Shastri Bhawan, New Delhi.

United Nations. 2002. Report by United Nations Secretary-General Kofi Annan released at the Second World Assembly on Ageing. Madrid, Spain, April 8–12. Published by the UN Department of Public Information DPI/2264, March.

Ushasree, S. and S. Azmal Basha. 1999. "Domestic abuse among the elderly". *Indian Journal of Gerontology* 13(3 and 4), pp. 99–104.

Vaithi, Savithri. 1996. "Elder abuse", paper presented at the National Workshop on Elder Abuse, organized by the Centre for the Welfare of the Aged (CEWA), Madras, March 16–17.

Verma, C.D. 1996. "Unwanted both by kin and society". *The Hindustan Times*, June 9.

WHO/INPEA. 2002. Missing Voices Views of Older Persons on Elder Abuse. Geneva: World Health Organization. WHO/NMH/VIP/02.1 WHO/NMH/NPH/02.2

13 Health Care for the Elderly

Subrata Mukherjee and Jean-Frédéric Levesque

The state of Kerala, in South India, is known for its remarkable achievements in the field of health and human development. Over a few decades, it has been able to reduce its levels of mortality to lower levels than other Indian states. It is often compared to other countries such as Sri Lanka and Costa Rica for having reached high levels of human development despite low levels of income (Franke and Chasin, 1992; Thankappan and Valiathan, 1998; Saradamma et al., 2000). Kerala has a life expectancy above 70 years and an infant mortality rate of 16 per thousand live births. It is comparable to many upper middle income countries, such as Argentina and Mauritius, in terms of life expectancy, infant mortality rate, and total fertility rate (World Bank, 2001).

Kerala is also seen as presenting lesser inequality between social groups than other Indian states (Drèze and Sen, 2002). Observers have suggested that this more equalitarian status is the result of the socialistic orientation of former governments and rulers resulting in land reforms and various public programmes (Panikar and Soman, 1975; Caldwell et al., 1983). The emphasis on primary education and on primary health care has resulted in the achievement of high levels of literacy and widespread access to maternal and child care services (Dreze and Sen, 1995; Kumar 1993). Kerala now has a highly literate, and *health literate* population, playing an active role in politics and public affairs and adopting hygienic practices (Shah and Rani, 2003; Kannan, 1999). Yet, recent assessment also suggests that Kerala presents the highest level of self-perceived morbidity, an ageing population and the highest level of private health care service utilization among Indian states (NSSO, 2006).

However, the state has been drawing attention of the researchers in recent years for what is called its second-generation problems such as educated unemployment, quality of education and problems of the elderly. Especially the situations of low mortality and low fertility have resulted into the ageing of Kerala society. Kerala now has the highest proportion of the elderly among major Indian states with 10.6 per cent of its population above 60 years of age in urban areas and 11.5 per cent in rural areas, compared to Indian averages respectively of 6.6 per cent and 7.0 per cent in urban and rural areas (Government of India, 2002; NSSO, 2006). Not much is known about the specific utilization pattern of the elderly in Kerala.

The chronic non-communicable diseases (CNCD) are emerging as a main cause of ill-health in South Asia. They now contribute to 53 per cent of deaths and 44 per cent of disability-adjusted life-years lost (Reddy et al., 2005). Almost half of the adult burden of disease in South Asia is attributable to CNCD and they occur at a younger age than in developed countries. Increase in life expectancy at birth – 63 years in South Asia – ageing of the population, and urbanization modifying social and environmental aspects of life are among the suggested factors related to this emergence of CNCD (World Bank, 2004). In addition, the traditional socio-economic gradients are changing with an increase in prevalence of risk factors, chronic illness and higher vulnerability to their detrimental effects among the poor (Ghaffar et al., 2004).

The prevalence of hypertension lies around 20–40 per cent and 12–17 per cent in urban and rural adults respectively. Dyslipidemia is also prevalent and suffers from a lack of detection. The prevalence of coronary heart disease is estimated at 3–4 per cent in rural areas and 8–10 per cent in urban areas (Reddy et al., 2005). Related to this is the prevalence of type II diabetes, estimated at 11.8 per cent and 3.8 per cent in urban and rural India (Reddy et al., 2005). Other non-communicable chronic diseases such as cancer and asthma are also rising problems. The main reasons of hospitalizations in India were infectious causes (21%), heart diseases and hypertensive disorders (11%), injuries (9%), cancers (3%), while psychiatric conditions were reported as main type of ailment in 0.6 per cent of cases (NSSO, 2006).

In Kerala, chronic conditions, such as type II diabetes, hypertension and coronary heart diseases are rising, alongside risk factors such as obesity, a sedentary lifestyle, elevated serum lipids and smoking (Kutty et al., 2000; Zachariah et al., 2003; Joseph et al., 2000; Boutayeb and Boutayeb, 2005). These chronic diseases are not restricted to the richer segments of populations since the poor show a strong prevalence and high rates of complications for many of these conditions (Ramachandran et al., 2002). These chronic diseases affect particularly the elderly population.

While public health care has traditionally been strong in Kerala, compared to other states, the public sector has not kept up with the growing demand for health care in recent years (Kumar, 1993; Nabae, 2003) and concerns have been expressed about its capacity to address the specific needs of the ageing population (Sureshkumar and Rajagopal, 1996; Bollini et al., 2004; Purohit, 2001). Recent decades have seen a considerable growth in private facilities in Kerala, so much that these now outstrip government facilities in number and in the provision of high-tech equipment. In Kerala, the private sector is prominent as it concentrates the large majority of the state's doctors (86%) and hospitals (82%); furthermore, 58% of hospital beds are in the private rather than in the public sector (Kutty et al., 2000; Varatharajan et al., 2002). The specific utilization of public and private facilities by the elderly in Kerala has not been assessed.

This chapter aims at understanding the specific patterns and consequences of utilization of health care services of the elderly in Kerala. The specific objectives of this chapter are as follow: (i) to understand the pattern of reported prevalence of illness among the elderly; and (ii) to understand the pattern of utilization of health care by the elderly in contrast to non-elderly. The chapter is divided into six sections including the present section. Section 2 briefly describes the methodology and data sources. Section 3 presents the pattern of reported prevalence of illness among elderly and non-elderly. Sections 4 and 5 present the empirical evidences on the utilization health care by the elderly and non-elderly population for outpatient care (section 4) and inpatient care services (section 5). Section 6 summarises the discussion and makes a few concluding remarks.

Methodology and Data Sources

For the purpose of this analysis, we have used the unit-record data from National Sample Survey 60th round for the state of Kerala. This survey was conducted during January-June 2004. It provides with population-based sample of urban and rural population in the state and employed a stratified sampling strategy. For Kerala, the survey provides information on illness and health care seeking behaviour of 13,333 individual coming from 2,829 households. The number of the elderly –

those aged of 60 years old or above – and non-elderly individuals in the sample are 1,766 and 11,567 respectively. All analyses were weighted to take into account the clustered sampling design.

The questionnaire employed covers a wide-range of demographic and health aspects and details about health care utilization for outpatient care (in the last 15 days) and inpatient care services (last 365 days). With regard to socio-economic status, NSS surveys provide a detailed assessment of household consumption expenditure per capita. To examine the variations in health care utilization pattern of the elderly and non-elderly across economic status, we have divided the population into per capita consumption expenditure quintiles (PCCE quintiles). For the purpose of this study, the bottom 30 per cent of the population according to PCCE have been considered as being *poor* while the top 10 per cent of the population were considered *rich* for comparison. Table 13.1 shows the range, median values and proportion of the Elderly by per capita consumption expenditure quintiles. From this table, we notice the important ranges among the poorest and richest quintiles, the increasing median expenditure and a slight increase in the proportion the elderly among richer segments.

Table 13.1 ***Select Summary Statistics for the Expenditure Quintiles***

PCCE Quintiles	*PCCE Range (Rs)*		*Median PCCE (Rs)*	*Percentage of elderly*
	Min	Max		
0–20	48	462	389	10.6
20–40	463	585	517	10.9
40–60	585	750	667	10.8
60–80	750	1000	864	11.3
80–100	1015	10875	1400	12.7

Source: Estimated from the unit-record NSS 60th round data

NSS classifies all households into a few occupational categories based on households' major source of income. Households in the rural sector are classified into five categories: *self-employed in agriculture, self-employed in non-agriculture, agricultural labour, other labour* and *others.* Similarly, households in the urban sector are classified into four categories: *self-employed, regular wage or salaried, casual labour* and *others.* When considered together all households in the rural and urban sector can be classified into four mutually exclusive categories: *labour, self-employed, regular wage or salaried* and *others*. The mean and median per capita consumption expenditure and percentage of total and the elderly population by occupational categories are presented in Table 13.2. From this table, we see that *labour* is the poorest class, followed by *self-employed*, while regular wage or salaried is the richest class. In terms of percentage population share, *labour* and *self-employed* categories are almost comparable. However, *self-employed* class accounts for the highest percentage of the elderly population. Although *regular wage or salaried* is the richest class, it accounts for only 7.2 per cent of the total population and 6.3 per cent of the elderly population. The *labour* and *self-employed* class together account for more than 70 per cent of the total population.

Table 13.2 ***Per Capita Household Consumption Expenditure (PCCE) and Population Share of Different Household Occupational Categories in Kerala***

Household occupational categories	*Per capita consumption expenditure*		*Share in*	
	Mean	Median	Total population	Old population
Labour	667	585	39,2	31,2
Self-employed	952	783	37,5	43,0
Regular wage/salaried	1438	1300	7,2	6,3
Others	1027	858	16,1	19,5

Source: Estimated from the unit-record NSS 60th round data.

For health expenditure data, we make a distinction between direct expenditure (medical cost) and indirect expenditure (access cost). The *medical cost* is the sum of all expenditure that an individual incurs at the health care facility for doctor's service, medicines, diagnostic tests etc, while *access cost* is the sum of monetary and non-monetary cost of accessing care, excluding the direct costs.

In order to control for the severity of illness - a known determinant of health care services utilization and level of expenditure – we have considered the presence of any days being confined to bed (bedridden) and duration of hospital stays in our analyses. This enabled us to disentangle the effect of severity of morbidity from other individual characteristics and assess the specific associations of age in multiple analyses.

Descriptive statistics and bivariate analyses were complemented with logistic regression models were developed using STATA 9.0 software. The outpatient care analysis consisted in two separate logistic regressions, the first one of utilization vs non-utilization in face of reported illness, the second being about utilizing a public vs private source of outpatient care. The inpatient care analysis consisted in a logistic regression of public vs private hospitalization and a linear regression of total health care expenditure for hospitalization. Reasons reported for utilizing a private facility complement the reported results.

Reported Morbidity

The number of persons reporting an ailment during a 15 days period in India stands at 91 per thousand persons. This is clearly higher than the previous estimates of 55 seen in 1995–96. In Kerala this cumulated prevalence now stands at 240 per thousand persons in urban areas and 255 per thousands in rural areas (NSSO, 2006). It was previously of 88 per thousand persons in previous estimates, disaggregated into 27 for chronic ailment and 61 for acute ailments per thousand persons (1995–96). Reported morbidity are approximately twice as high in Kerala compared to other south Indian states. Its reported rate of 100 commencing ailment per 1,000 persons in urban areas is twice the incidence reported for the second highest state, Maharashtra (NSSO, 2006).

Figure 13.1 ***Reported Prevalence of Illness among the Elderly and Non-elderly Population across PCCE Quintiles, in the last 15 Days***

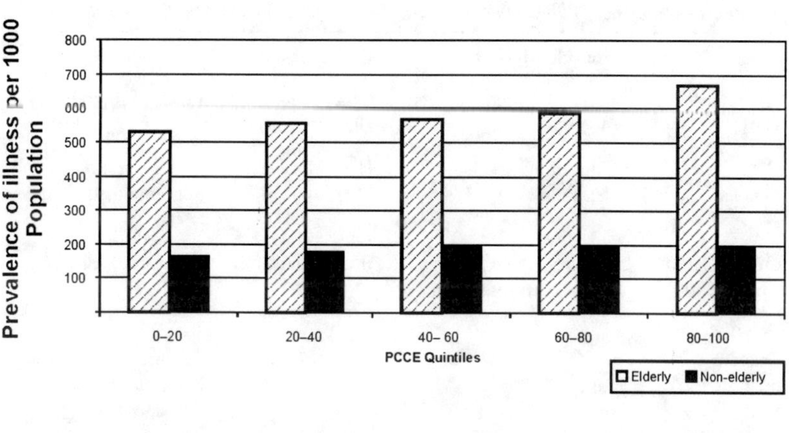

The pattern of reported prevalence of illness of the elderly and non-elderly population across economic classes provides a backdrop for understanding their health care utilization pattern. The reported prevalence of illness across PCCE quintiles is depicted in Figure 13.1. From this figure, we can see that, as expected, for any given economic status, the reported prevalence of illness is substantially higher for the elderly population compared to non-elderly population. It is in fact higher than 50 per cent of, elderly reporting any ailments during a 15 days period in Kerala for every income groups. These results must reflect the prevalence of chronic illnesses among the elderly. Table 13.3 shows the five most prevalent diseases among the elderly and non-elderly in our sample. Despite limitations in the survey – very high levels of *other diagnosed ailments* are reported – the contrast is interesting. Four of the five most reported diseases for the elderly are related to chronic ailments with heart disease and diabetes also topping the list with regards to causes of hospitalizations. Infectious disorders are – as expected – more prevalent among non elderly.

In addition, Figure 13.1 reveals that, although the reported prevalence of illness shows increases with economic status, the gradient is stronger for the elderly population compared to the non-elderly population. Assuming that individuals with lower income show less awareness about health and health care and poor access to health care and therefore systematically understate their health status, these results are underestimates of true differentials in health in Kerala.

Table 13.3 ***The Highest Five Prevalent Illness for the Elderly and Non-Elderly***

Reported morbidity per 1000 population		*Hospitalization per 1000 population*	
Elderly	Non-elderly	Elderly	Non-elderly
Hypertension (121)	Fever of unknown origin (48)	Other diagnosed ailments (38)	Fever of unknown origin (22)
Disorder of joints and bones (96)	Other diagnosed elements (37)	Heart disease (36)	Other diagnosed ailments (19)
Other diagnosed ailments (90)	Respiratory including ear/nose/throat ailments (35)	Bronchial asthma (26)	Fractures/poisoning (10)
Diabetes mellitus (86)	Disorder of joints and bones (15)	Diabetes mellitus (22)	Respiratory including ear/nose/throat ailments (7)
Heart disease (55)	Hypertension (10)	Fever of unknown origin (22)	Diarrhoea/dysentery (5)

Source: Estimated from the unit-record NSS 60th round data.

Utilization of Outpatient Care

Kerala has traditionally reported high levels of treatment in face of illness among Indian states. Results from our analysis confirms this with more than 88 per cent of illness receiving medical treatments in the last 15 days. The percentage of treated illness for the elderly and non-elderly population across PCCE quintiles is presented in Figure 13.2. The percentage of treated illness tends to increase with economic status for the elderly. However, such trend is not clear for the non-elderly. To examine this point more closely, we present the percentage of treated illness of poor and rich elderly and non-elderly in Table 13.4. The table shows that percentage of treated illness is much higher for the rich elderly compared to the poor elderly. This difference is not there when poor non-elderly and rich non-elderly are compared.

Figure 13.2 ***Percentage of Treated Illness for the Elderly and Non-Elderly Population***

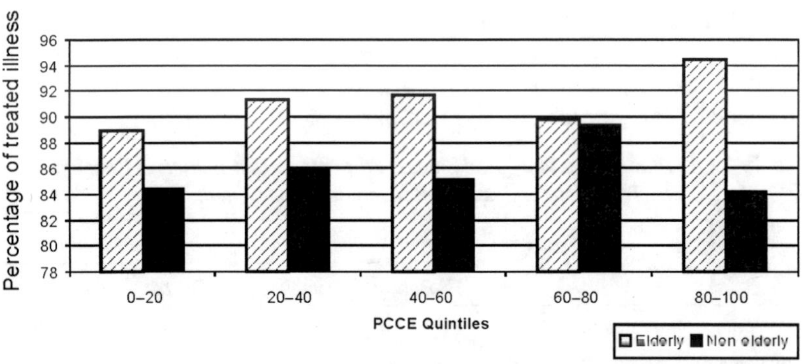

Intuitively, when an individual does not seek health care, there could be two possible reasons for such behaviour. First, when the individual perceives that expected impact of health care on health is not enough to compensate for the loss of consumption of non-health care goods, individual may not seek health care. This can happen when the individual does not perceive the illness as a serious one. Secondly, when the sacrifice of the consumption of non-health care goods is not feasible, the individual may delay seeking health care, go for informal care or may not seek health care at all.

Information collected in NSS 60th round on 'reasons for no treatment' helps us to understand the reasons behind individuals' decision of no health care. The percentage distribution of non-treated illness by reasons shows that except for the rich elderly, the reason illness not serious enough appears to be the major reason for not seeking health care. But this is individuals' perception about seriousness of illness and need not be the actual seriousness of illness if the seriousness was measured in an objective manner (say clinical test). It is not difficult to understand that an individual's assessment about the seriousness of an illness is highly influenced by her awareness and access to health care.

The reasons for no health care can be reclassified based on our conceptual framework. Absence of any facility in the neighbourhood and long waiting time imply that the household (not necessarily the ill individual alone) needs to spend longer time to utilise health care, in addition to other monetary expenditure associated with seeking health care. If the employment nature of the household does not allow enough time to utilise health care without sacrificing income, then longer time also implies higher non-monetary access cost. So both *no facility available* and *long waiting* imply higher access cost. Financial reason basically imply higher direct price. So we can reclassify the reasons for no treatment into three mutually exclusive categories: higher access cost, higher direct price and other reasons. It is important to know that higher direct price as a reason no treatment is higher for the elderly (especially for the rich elderly) compared to the non-elderly.

Table 13.4 ***Percentage of treated Illness, Percentage Distribution of Reasons for no Treatment and Loss of Household Income (INR)***

	Poor		*Rich*	
	Elderly	*Non-elderly*	*Elderly*	*Non-elderly*
Percentage of treated illness	89.3	85.4	95.9	85.6
Reasons for no treatment				
No facility available	—	1.6	—	—
Lack of faith	6.5	1.6	—	2.9
Long waiting	0.0	0.0	—	—
Financial reasons	36.7	32.6	52.8	0.7
Ailment not serious	37.0	54.7	19.1	81.6
Others	19.8	9.4	28.1	14.8
Reasons for no treatment (reclassified)				
High access cost	—	1.6	—	—
High medical cost	36.7	32.6	52.8	0.7
Other reasons	63.3	65.8	47.2	99.3
Loss of household income (Rs)	62	86	15	74

Source: Estimated from the unit-record NSS 60th round data.

The loss of household income per illness episode is presented in Table 13.4. As expected rich loose less income due to illness compared to the poor. Since the average income of the rich class is much higher than the poor class, average loss of income of the rich as a percentage of their average income is substantially lower than that of the poor. On an average a household looses less income when an elderly falls sick compared to a situation when a non-elderly falls sick. But it is interesting to note that a poor household looses substantial income not only when a non-elderly member falls sick but also when an elderly member falls sick. The difference in average loss of household income due to illness between elderly and non-elderly is noticeably lower when we compare such difference between rich elderly and rich non-elderly. In other words, poor households tend to loose income more even as a result of an illness of an elderly member. This could be because of the reasons that in poor households along with non-elderly productive age group, elderly are also important earning members. In other words, poor households' incomes crucially depend on the health status of the elderly as well.

Table 13.5 ***Logistic Regression Results of Utilization of Medical care in Case of Reported Illness (n = 2,990)***

	Coefficient	*Odds ratio*	*p value*
Intercept	1.7943		
Severity of illness (REF = not bedridden)			
Bedridden	0.6462	1.9083	0.005
Per capita consumption expenditure			
Age group (REF = 0–59)	0.0001	1.0001	0.502
60 years and above	0.5973	1.8171	0.000
Sex (REF = Female)			
Male	–0.2093	0.8111	0.130
Household occupational category (REF = Casual labour)			
Self-employed	–0.0817	0.9216	0.595
Regular wage/salaried	–0.1894	0.8275	0.531

Note: Weighted logistic regression where weight is inverse of household probability of selection. The occupational category others is excluded because of multicollinearity problem.

Source: Estimated from NSS 60th round unit-record data.

We estimated a logistic regression to examine the association between an ill individual's utilization and non-utilization of health care and a set of important independent variables. The result of the logistic regression is presented in Table 13.5. It is found that age and severity of illness are significantly associated with an ill individual's decision to utilise health care. In fact after controlling for severity of illness and economic status, an ill elderly individual has 1.8 more times propensity to utilise health care compared to the non-elderly people. Economic status, sex and household occupational categories are not significantly associated with an ill individual's decision to utilise health care.

Once an ill individual decides to utilise health care, she faced the problem of choice between alternative health care providers. To an individual each health care provider represents a particular combination of quality, direct price and access costs. The individual chooses the health care provider who is expected to give her maximum utility. Since it is not possible to examine empirically the effects of quality, direct price and access cost on individual's choice of outpatient care providers given the type of data we have, we will rather attempt to present some direct and indirect evidences which would highlight the role that quality, access cost and direct price play in an individual's choice of health care providers.

Table 13.6 ***Percentage of Treatment from Government Sources and Reasons for not Utilization of Government Facilities***

	Poor		*Rich*	
	Elderly	*Non-Elderly*	*Elderly*	*Non-Elderly*
Any treatment received from govt. sources	44.9	49.9	17.6	15.7
Reasons for non-utilization of government facilities				
Government doctor/facility too far	19.0	18.8	9.1	14.0
Not satisfied with medical treatment by govt. doctor/facility	25.8	32.7	40.6	36.0
Long waiting	14.1	8.8	23.0	22.0
Required specific services not available	10.1	12.7	12.2	9.58
Others	31.0	27.0	14.2	18.5

Source: Estimated from NSS 60th round unit-record data.

The percentage of illness episodes for which health care was sought from government sources is presented in Table 13.6. The table shows that poor elderly utilize government facilities less than the poor non-elderly, but the rich elderly utilize government facilities more than the rich non-elderly. The same table also presents the reasons for non-utilization of government facilities. Reasons for non-utilization of government facilities relate more around access reasons for the poor, with no difference between elderly and non-elderly while it relates more to quality of care related reasons for the rich.

The median direct price and monetary access cost per treated illness for the elderly and non-elderly population are presented in Table 13.7. On an average the elderly spend more than the non-elderly for treatment of a single illness episode. Since the elderly people suffer mostly from chronic illness, which require treatment for long duration, the monetary cost of treatment is expected to be higher for them.

As far as monetary cost per illness episode is concerned, there is a huge difference between the rich elderly and the rich non-elderly. However such difference is very small in the poor class. If we assume that there is least discrimination against the elderly in the rich class as far as spending on their health is concerned, then small difference in monetary cost of treatment between the poor-elderly and the poor non-elderly could be an indication of discrimination against the former. In other words, small difference in monetary cost of treatment between elderly and non-elderly among the poor compared to that among the rich could mean a restriction of spending on needs of the elderly among the poor.

Table 13.7 ***Median Direct Price and Monetary Access Cost per Treated Illness for the Elderly and Non-Elderly People in Kerala (last 15 days)***

	Poor		*Rich*	
	Elderly	*Non-elderly*	*Elderly*	*Non-elderly*
Medical costs	100	85	225	110
Monetary access cost	20	10	15	15

Source: Estimated from the unit-record NSS 60th round data.

To understand people's choice between government and private providers for outpatient care we have estimated a logistic regression. The results of the logistic regression are presented in Table 13.8. The table shows that the variables economic status, sex, household occupational category are significantly associated with choice of health care providers. Higher economic status and non-casual labour categories are associated with increased probability of utilizing a private provider. It is important to note that choice of the provider is not significantly associated with age group (such as elderly and non-elderly), sex. Severity of illness, although it tends to be associated with an increase probability in private utilization does not reach statistical significance level in our multiple regressions.

Table 13.8 ***Logisitic Regression Results of Private Source of Outpatient Care (n = 2,528).***

	Coefficient	*Odds ratio*	*p value*
Intercept	–0.2886		
Severity of illness (REF = not bedridden)			
Bedridden	0.2837	1.3280	0.059
Per capita consumption expenditure	0.0006	1.0006	0.008
Age group (REF = 0–59)			
60 years and above	0.1164	1.1235	0.284
Sex (REF = Female)			
Male	–0.1750	0.8394	0.095
Household occupational category (REF = Casual labour)			
Self-employed	0.6249	1.8680	0.000
Regular wage/salaried	0.9772	2.6571	0.000

Note: Weighted logistic regression where weight is inverse of household probability of selection. The occupational category others is excluded because of multicollinearity problem.

Source: Estimated from NSS 60th round unit-record data.

Utilization of Inpatient Care

The state of Kerala presents the highest rates of hospitalization among Indian states (NSSO 2006). The rate of utilization of inpatient care (per 1,000 population) by the elderly and non-elderly population across PCCE quintiles are presented in Figure 13.3. We make three observations from this figure. First, the rate of utilization of inpatient care is much higher for the elderly compared to the non-elderly for all economic status. Second, except for the fourth quintile, the rate of utilization of inpatient care shows as increase with economic status.[1] Third, utilization of inpatient care shows a strong gradient with increasing income class among the elderly but almost no variation among non-elderly. This suggests that – assuming a similar relationship between need for care and income among the elderly and the non-elderly – hospitalization of the poor elderly could be restricted.

The percentage of inpatient care from government sources (separately for elderly and non-elderly) across economic status is presented in Figure 13.4. We make two observations from the figure. First, dependence of the elderly on government facilities is marginally higher compared to the non-elderly. Second, dependence of people on government facilities for inpatient care is quite high for first four quintiles without any systematic fall, and then it substantially falls in the fifth quintile (the richest class). In other words, no significant difference is found between the elderly and the non-elderly in the choice of inpatient care and income gradient in choice is not very clear.

Figure 13.3 ***The Rate of Utilization of Inpatient care per 1000 Population***

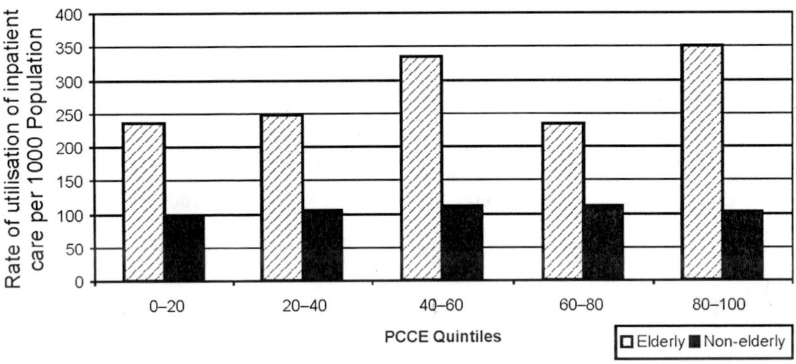

Figure 13.4 ***Percentage of Inpatient Care from Government Sources***

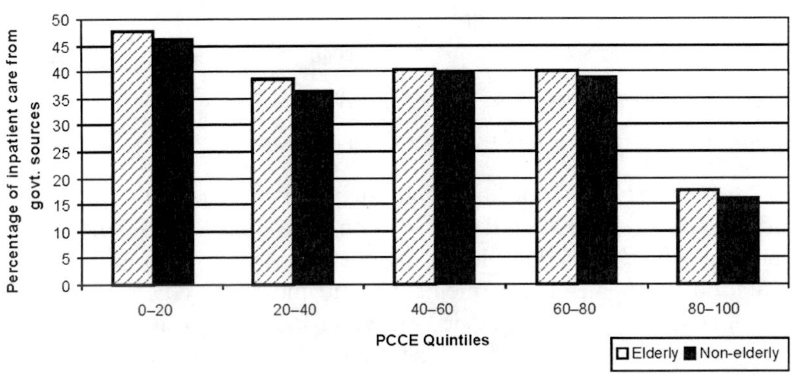

The median monetary cost incurred by the elderly and the non-elderly population per inpatient care is presented in Table 13.9. As expected the monetary cost of private inpatient care is substantially higher than that of government care. As far as the non-elderly are concerned, there is not much difference between total monetary price paid by the rich and by the poor. Surprisingly, total monetary price paid by the rich elderly at government facilities is much higher than that at the private facilities. The rich elderly who utilized government facilities for inpatient care also incurred higher monetary expenditure compared to their non-elderly counter-part. Probably the rich elderly who utilized government facilities for inpatient care suffered from long-term chronic illnesses, which would prove too costly at private hospitals.

Table 13.9 ***Median Direct Price, Monetary Access Cost and Total Monetary Cost Per Inpatient Care for the Poor and Rich Elderly***

	Poor		*Rich*	
	Government	*Private*	*Government*	*Private*
Elderly				
Direct price	700	2220	5900	3550
Monetary access cost	100	50	300	150
Total monetary price	830	2255	7090	3950
Non-elderly				
Direct price	510	1850	850	3188
Monetary access cost	100	87	60	150
Total monetary price	670	2012	860	3188
Combined				
Direct price	510	1872	1500	3188
Monetary access cost	100	87	100	150
Total monetary price	680	2040	1599	3550

Note: Total monetary price = direct price + monetary access cost.

Source: Estimated from the unit-record NSS 60th round data.

The average loss of household income per hospitalization case is presented in Table 13.10. Expectedly, on an average a household looses more income when a non-elderly member is hospitalized compared to a situation when an elderly member is hospitalized. When an elderly member is hospitalized a poor household looses more income than a rich household even in absolute amount. In poor households the elder person also contributes to household income. So when an elderly person from a poor household gets hospitalized, the household looses substantial number of working hours and in poor households compensating for the lost working hours is difficult. However, when a non-elderly member is hospitalized, poor and rich household loose almost comparable amount of income in absolute terms. Since the average income of a poor household is much lower than that of a rich household, loss as a percentage of income must be very high for the poor household compared to the rich.

Table 13.10 ***Average Loss of Household Income (Rs) per Hospitalization Episode.***

Economic class	*Elderly*	*Non-elderly*
Poor	214	640
Rich	166	646

Source: Estimated from the unit-record NSS 60th round data.

To understand the association between people's choice between government and private inpatient care and a few important individual/household level characteristics we have estimated a logistic regression. The independent variables that we have considered are PCCE (as a proxy for economic status), household's occupational category, age group, sex and duration of stay in the hospital (as a proxy for severity of illness). Economic status and household occupational categories are positively associated with choice favouring private hospital. Gender and age group do not show any significant choice favouring utilization of private hospital. If we assume duration of stay in hospital as a proxy for severity of illness, then it seems that severity reduces the probability of utilization of private hospital.

Table 13.11 ***Logisitic Regression Results of Private Source of Inpatient Care (n = 1,551)***

	Coefficient	*Odds ratio*	*p value*
Intercept	–0.0693		
Duration of hospital stay	–0.0455	0.9555	0.000
Per capita consumption expenditure	0.0008	1.0008	0.000
Age group (REF = 0–59)			
60 years and above	–0.0689	0.9334	0.636
Sex (REF = Female)			
Male	0.1799	1.1971	0.147
Household occupational category (REF = Casual labour)			
Self-employed	0.6876	1.9890	0.000
Regular wage/salaried	0.6437	1.9035	0.006

Note: Weighted logistic regression where weight is inverse of household probability of selection. The household occupational category others is excluded because of multicollinearity problem.

Source: Estimated from NSS 60th round unit-record data.

Discussion and Conclusion

Our results confirm high levels of reporting of ailments and high rates of hospitalization among the elderly in the state of Kerala. Age is a determinant of getting outpatient care in the face of illness in Kerala, controlling for other important factors. This could not be assessed for hospitalization because of the nature of the survey. This is in line with the tradition of consulting medical facilities in need for care present in Kerala. Yet, the proportion of utilization in face of need among the elderly is strongly associated with income in Kerala, as measured by the gradient of utilization with increasing PCCE in our study, controlling for severity of illness. This first analysis of a population-based survey reporting disparities in utilization among poor and rich elderly is a cause for concern in Kerala. This question should be tackled by more complete assessments in further studies.

A further observation from our analyses is the fact that elderly status is not associated with utilization of private and public facilities for both outpatient and inpatient services in Kerala. The disparities between these sectors is mostly taken up by economic related variables such as PCCE and household occupational status, the poor resorting more to public facilities for their care than richer segments of the population. The fact that the elderly people do not differ from the non-elderly with this regards could suggest that individual choices of the elderly are strongly influenced by household patterns of consumption of health care.

The expenditure for health care in Kerala is higher for the elderly both in outpatient and inpatient care. This goes in line with higher prevalence of long-term chronic illnesses among the aged. Interestingly, expenditure for the aged coming from wealthier background in the public sector are even higher than in the private sector. This could come from the fact that hospitalization for chronic illnesses for the non-poor elderly might prove too expensive in Kerala in the private sector in Kerala. Another hypothesis is that for certain chronic ailments, the prospect of consulting in medical colleges – benefiting from specialist services and invasive technologies – could be a preferred option, private care being reserved for other more common ailments. Further studies are needed to clarify this.

Interestingly, illness among the aged is associated with loss of income in Kerala, albeit less than in the case of non-elderly members. This is especially true for poor households. Could it be that elderly are economically productive, especially in poor households, or the result of the fact that the poor elderly consult more in the public, known for longer waiting times?

Our approach is to study the utilization pattern of people in two ways: studying their utilization – non-utilization and studying their choice of health care providers. We study the health care utilization pattern of people separately for the elderly and the non-elderly population. It is well documented in the literature that apart from population characteristics two factors, which determine the health care utilization pattern, are price and quality of health care. We define both the quality and price of health care from individual perspectives. Defined in this way, quality is the expected ability of care to produce the highest possible outcome according to individual's evaluation.

Note

1. Such exceptional pattern in the utilization in the fourth PCCE quintile is also observed in case of utilization of outpatient care.

References

Bhutta, Z., S. Nundy and K. Abbasi. 2004. "Is there hope for South Asia. Yes, if we can replicate the models of Kerala and Sri Lanka". *BMJ* 3 April, 328: 777–778.

Bhutta, Z.A., I. Gupta, H. deSilva, D. Manandhar, S. Awasthi, S.M. Moazzem and M.A. Salam. 2004. "Maternal and child health: is South Asia ready for change?" *British Medical Journal* (*BMJ*), 3 April, 328: 816–9.

Bollini, P., C. Venkateswaran and K. Sureshkumar. 2004. "Palliative care in Kerala, India: a model for resource-poor settings". *Onkologie* 27 April (2): 138–42.

Boutayeb, A. and S. Boutayeb. 2005. "The burden of non-communicable diseases in developing countries". *International Journal for Equity in Health* 4: 2. doi: 10.1186/1475–9276–4–2.

Caldwell, J.C., P.H. Reddy and P. Caldwell. 1983. "The Social Component of Mortality Decline: An Investigation in South India Employing Alternative Methodology". *Population Studies* 37: 185–205.

Drèze, J. and A. Sen. 1995. "India: Economic development and social opportunity". New Delhi: Oxford University Press, p. 306.

——. 2002. India: Development and Participation". New Delhi: Oxford University Press, p. 540.

Franke, R.W. and B.H. Chasin. 1992. "Kerala state, India: Radical reform as development". *International Journal of Health Services* 22(1): 139–156.

Ghaffar, A., K. Srinath Reddy and M. Singhi. 2004. "Burden of non-communicable diseases in South Asia". *BMJ* 3 April, 328: 807–810.

Government of India. 2002. "National Human Development Report". 2001. Planning commission, Government of India, March.

Joseph, A., V.R. Kutty and C.R. Soman. 2000. "High risk for coronary heart disease in Thiruvananthapuram city: A study of serum lipids and other risk factors". *Indian Heart J.* January–February, 52(1): 29–35.

Kannan, K.P. 1999. "Poverty alleviation as advancing basic human capabilities: Kerala's achievements compared". Working Paper No. 294, Centre for Development Studies, Thiruvanthapuram, India, May.

Kumar, B.G. 1993. "Low Mortality and High Morbidity in Kerala Reconsidered". *Population and Development Review* 19(1): 103–21.

Kutty, V.R., C.R. Soman, A. Joseph, R. Pisharody and K. Vijayakumar. 2000. "Type 2 diabetes in southern Kerala: variation in prevalence among geographic divisions within a region". *Natl Med J India* November–December, 13(6): 284–6.

Nabae, K. 2003. "The Health Care System in Kerala: Its Past Accomplishments and New Challenges". *Journal of the National Institute of Public Health* 52(2): 140–145.

NSSO. 2006. Morbidity, Health care and the Condition of the Aged. NSS 60th round. January–June 2004. National Sample Survey Organisation, Ministry of Statistics and Programme Implementation, Government of India, March.

Panikar, P.G.K. and C.R. Soman. 1975. "Health Status of Kerala: The Paradox of Economic Backwardness and Health Development". Centre for Development Studies, Thiruvanthapuram, Kerala, India.

Purohit, B.C. 2001. "Private initiatives and policy options: recent health system experience in India". *Health Policy and Planning* 16(1): 87–97.

Ramachandran, A., C. Snehalatha, V. Vijay and H. King. 2002. "Impact of poverty on the prevalence of diabetes and its complications in urban southern India". *Diabet Med.* Feb. 19(2): 130–5.

Reddy, K.S., B. Shah, C. Varghese and A. Ramadoss 2005. "Responding to the threat of chronic diseases in India". *The Lancet* 366: 1746–51.

Saradamma, R.D., N. Higginbotham and M. Nichter. 2000. "Social factors influencing the acquisition of antibiotics without prescription in Kerala State, South India". *Social Science and Medicine* 50: 891–903.

Shah, S. and M. Rani. 2003. "Worlds apart: Why are Kerala and Uttar Pradesh so different in their human development outcomes?" Background paper for the World Development Report 2004, Making the Services Work for Poor People. The World Bank, Washington, p. 8.

Sureshkumar, K. and M.R. Rajagopal. 1996. "Palliative care in Kerala. Problems at presentation in 440 patients with advanced cancer in a south Indian state". *Palliat Med.* Oct., 10(4): 293–8.

Thankappan, K.R. and M.S. Valiathan. 1998. "Health at low cost: the Kerala model". *Lancet* 351: 1274–1275.

Varatharajan, D., R. Sadanandan, K.R. Thankappan and Nair V. Mohnan. 2002. "Idle capacity in resource strapped government hospitals in Kerala: Size, distribution and determining factors. Thiruvananthapuram: Achuta Menon Centre for Health Science Studies", Sree Chitra Tirunal Institute for Medical Sciences and Technology.

World Bank. 2001. India, Raising the sights: Better Health Systems for India's Poor. Health, Nutrition, Population

Sector Unit, India: South Asian Region, November 3. World Bank. 2004. *India at a glance*. The World Bank group.

Zachariah, M.G., K.R. Thankappan, S.C. Alex, P.S. Sarma and R.S. Vasan. 2003. "Prevalence, correlates, awareness, treatment, and control of hypertension in a middle-aged urban population in Kerala". *Indian Heart Journal,* May–June, 55(3): 245–51.

Contributors

D. Dalus, M.D., Superintendent, Thiruvananthapuram Medical College, Thiruvananthapuram, Kerala

A.B. Dey, M.D., Professor & Chief of Geriatric Services, Department of Medicine, All India Institute of Medical Sciences, New Delhi. Formerly, President of both Association on Gerontology and Indian Academy of Geriatrics.

I.S. Gambhir, M.D., Professor and Head, Division of Geriatrics, Professor, Department of Medicine, I.M.S., Banaras Hindu University, Varanasi, Uttar Pradesh.

S. Irudaya Rajan, Ph.D., Chair Professor, Research Unit on International Migration, Centre for Development Studies, Thiruvananthapuram, India. He has published two books on ageing and completed five projects on various ageing related issues.

C. Shanthi Johnson, Ph.D., Professor, School of Nutrition and Dietetics, Acadia University, Wolfville, Nova Scotia, Canada. & Canadian Centre for Activity and Aging, Faculty of Health Sciences, The University of Western Ontario, London, Ontario, Canada.

Gareth R. Jones, Ph.D., Assistant Professor, Faculty of Health Sciences and the Canadian Centre for Activity and Aging, The University of Western Ontario, London, Ontario, Canada. Formerly, the Director of the Canadian Centre for Activity and Ageing.

Roy Abraham Kallivayalil, M.D., Professor and Head, Dept. of Psychiatry, Govt. Medical College, Thrissur, Kerala and Secretary General, SAARC Psychiatric Federation.

B. Krishnaswamy, M.D., Professor and Head, Department of Geriatric Medicine, Madras Medical College, Chennai. He is currently the President of the Indian Academy of Geriatrics.

Jean-Frédéric Levesque, M.D., Ph.D., Institut de sante publique du Quebec and Unite de internationale, Universite de Montreal, Canada

Arvind Mathur, M.D., Associate Professor, Department of Medicine, SN Medical College, Jodhpur, Rajasthan. Currently, he is the Editor of the *Journal of the Indian Academy of Geriatrics*, official publication of the Indian Academy of Geriatrics.

Subrata Mukherjee, Ph.D., Assistant Professor, Institute of Development Studies, Kolkata, India. Formerly, he was with Center for Development Studies, Thiruvananthapuram, Kerala.

V.S. Natarajan, M.D., Geriatric Physician and Chairman, Senior Citizens Bureau. Formerly Head, at Department of Geriatric Medicine, Madras Medical College, Chennai.

Seema Puri, Ph.D., Reader and Health, Department of Nutrition, Institute of Home Economics, Delhi University. She is board member of the Society for Gerontological Research, New Delhi.

Mala Kapur Shankardass, Ph.D., Reader, Department of Sociology, Maitreyi College, University of Delhi, and she is also the National Representative of International Network for Prevention of Elder Abuse (INPEA).

G.S. Shanthi, M.D., Assistant Professor, Geriatrician and Gynecologist, Department of Geriatric Medicine, Madras Medical College, Chennai. She is a member of the Association on Gerontology, India.

M.K. Thakur, Ph.D., Professor and Head, Department of Zoology, Banaras Hindu University, Varanasi, India. Currently, he is the President of the Association of Gerontology (India).

Index